A Body
Out of Balance

D0981424

A Body Out of Balance

Understanding
and Treating
Sjögren's
Syndrome

RUTH FREMES, M.A.
and
NANCY CARTERON, M.D., FACR

AVERY
a member of Penguin Group (USA) Inc.
New York

Most Avery books are available at special quantity discounts for bulk purchase for sales promotions, premiums, fund-raising, and educational needs. Special books or book excerpts also can be created to fit specific needs. For details, write Penguin Group (USA) Inc. Special Markets, 375 Hudson Street, New York, NY 10014.

a member of
Penguin Group (USA) Inc.
375 Hudson Street
New York, NY 10014
www.penguin.com

Library of Congress Cataloging-in-Publication Data

Fremes, Ruth, date.
A body out of balance : understanding and treating Sjögren's syndrome / Ruth Fremes and
Nancy Carteron.
p.   cm.
Includes bibliographical references and index.
ISBN 1-58333-172-7
1. Sjögren's syndrome—Popular works.   I. Carteron, Nancy.   II. Title.
RC647.5.S5F745   2003   2003052204
616.7'7—dc21

Printed in the United States of America
7   9   10   8

BOOK DESIGN BY TANYA MAIBORODA

Acknowledgments

THIS PROJECT HAD A LIFE OF ITS OWN AS WE WENT about drafting, writing, and correcting our manuscript. What began as a simple idea—"Let's write a book about Sjögren's syndrome"—became a fascinating process of discovery. It seemed that there was so much information waiting to be encountered, understood, and written about as we looked at the exciting field of autoimmunity in general and Sjögren's syndrome in particular. Our computers whizzed through the process with efficiency, presenting us with further insights and additions. As the writing came to a close, our friends and colleagues graciously agreed to help: to read our words, correct them, and add some insights of their own.

We owe a debt of gratitude to them all: Drs. Kenneth Fye, David Wofsy, Helen Emery, Amy Saltzman, Ricki Pollycove, Karen Oxford; our friends, Allan Grill, Clare Goodman, Carol Kirk, Pat Trumbull; and our families, who listened attentively as we talked ceaselessly about our project, deserve special accolades. A special thanks is due to Professor Zak Sabry, who, as always, encouraged and supported us while helping to make the nutrition information accessible for the reader.

We also wish to thank our patients and fellow Sjögren's sufferers, whose questions initiated this project and fueled it as it materialized.

To our male colleagues, we hope you will accept our gender preference in the body of the work. This reflects no bias—simply a convenience and ease of expression.

Our publishing associates deserve special mention. Agent Andrée Abecassis, old-time friend John Duff, and, always helpful and supportive, editor Kristen Jennings.

Thank you all.

*For our patients and friends with autoimmune disorders,
especially those for whom a diagnosis was long in coming*

and

*For our support group members, whose stories bring to light the dilemmas
faced by all those with Sjögren's syndrome.*

*It is our hope that information, creative problem solving,
and good treatment strategies will improve your quality of life today,
and new research will promise a true cure in the future.*

Contents

Foreword

THE CONCEPT OF PATIENTS WITH CHRONIC DIS-
eases as passive consumers of health care is changing. The new paradigm
looks to expert patients as partners with professionals in providing their
own health care. In no disease is this more important than for Sjögren's
syndrome. SjS is a disease in which patients need to identify important
symptoms involving many parts of the body. Patients must navigate
among multiple professionals who specialize in the eye, mouth, or joints
rather than having a complete "Sjögren's" doctor, and they have to select
among an array of over-the-counter medications in addition to prescription drugs. To successfully manage this disease, expert Sjögren's patients
must be created who are educated, informed, and empowered.

A Body Out of Balance: Understanding and Treating Sjögren's Syndrome
provides the information patients need to become experts. It will enable
them to understand how SjS may affect their own body, give them the as-
surance to seek the help they need, and provide them with the means to
cope with the inevitable symptoms, like fatigue, which may remain despite
the best of care. I urge all patients to read this book, refer to it often, and
then think of themselves as an expert patient. Should they also have the
urge to strike back at their disease, they can join the Sjögren's Syndrome
Foundation and join the fight against Sjögren's.

—ARTHUR I. GRAYZEL, M.D., MACR
Past President, Sjögren's Syndrome Foundation

Introduction
by Ruth Fremes, the Patient

"Exercise." "Live a normal life." "Try not to think about it." This advice rattled round in my head as I sat in the doctor's office and tried to make sense of his words while trying to ignore the tiredness, pain, dry eyes, and numb feet that overwhelmed me. Goodness knows I wanted to follow his prescription. I just couldn't seem to. Every effort was too much; every body movement hurt; every blink of an eye burned.

THAT WAS TWELVE YEARS AGO. BACK THEN, I WAS your average overachiever, busy with work and home. I had enrolled in graduate school to enter a new profession when the sudden appearance of vague, diffuse, debilitating symptoms intruded and sent me reeling from doctor to doctor. And it was then, after a series of inconclusive tests, that my then doctor advised me to just ignore whatever I thought I had—that I probably had a "collagen-vascular disease"—and dismissed me, saying that I "should get active and get on with my life." I left his office determined to try both exercise and normalcy. That the disease interfered with this treatment plan and my new career is not surprising.

During those twelve years, I underwent a series of unsatisfying experiments and tests, some intrusive, others worthless. I used palliatives like blepharitis drops for my stinging eyes, massage therapy for my aching joints, and Pilates treatment for my shrinking muscles. I endured gastrointestinal investigations, CT scans, MRIs, painful tests of my peripheral nerves, and, with the failure of all of these, psychotherapy for my depressed mood. The tests did show some abnormalities but nothing that could direct the doctor to a definitive diagnosis. I pined for something—anything—that would have a medical solution. Nothing came. Ironically, the more I was turned away from medicine's answer, the more I longed for it—and the more depressed I became.

Today I am diagnosed with Sjögren's syndrome and have an understanding of the disease and its activity in my body. The journey to diagnosis was strenuous. Learning to live with the disease has been disheartening. But that knowledge has finally brought me peace of mind.

For some, the road to diagnosis is smooth; for most, however, it is bumpy. There are many dead ends, detours, and false starts. It's a continuing process, but with diagnosis comes understanding and with understanding comes acceptance; with acceptance comes adjustment, and with that (and education) we have the ability to make judgments about care.

I wondered why SjS was so difficult to diagnose. With hindsight I realize that, for one thing, the symptoms are diffuse and ambiguous; they seem to mimic other conditions. They can look and feel like prolonged persistent flu or arthritis. The fatigue can easily be looked upon as a lack of sleep. Dry eyes can look like infectious conjunctivitis. A persistent cough can imitate a stubborn flu. When a patient presents herself to her family doctor with any or all of these symptoms, she will likely receive the diagnosis of anemia or malingering or mild depression.

To make matters worse, managed care has inserted itself into the doctor-patient relationship. Managed care with its controls, requirements, and time constraints pressures our doctors in ways that discourage thoughtful diagnoses.

Each of the symptoms of Sjögren's syndrome calls for a different medical specialty: ophthalmology for the eyes, oral medicine for the mouth, gastroenterology for the GI disturbances, neurology for the tingling nerves, and on and on. Since none of these specialties report to each other, it's not difficult to understand why an integrated picture of the patient is elusive.

These reasons conjoin to confound the process and seriously hinder effective health care for sufferers of chronic disease.

It's the wise family doctor who refers this kind of patient to a rheumatologist, for that's where she belongs. And that is how I began my steady road to recovery. When I found myself with a rheumatologist who was able to say, after a round of tests, "You're suffering from Sjögren's syndrome," I felt like shouting Hallelujah! Finally, a diagnosis!

While diagnosis is significant, it is simply the first step in the journey. I have found that just as I secure a treatment for one symptom, another equally bothersome one will intrude. But that is the nature of a chronic disease. It demands much of us. We must constantly reevaluate our health status in order to have the best possible quality of life.

I remember when I awakened to the realization that I had gone through all five stages of grief: from denial through anger; bargaining to depression, and finally acceptance. I had pretended I was the same as others when I was suffering. I had railed against the disease in private and in public as well. I sank into a numbing depression. And, finally, when nothing had changed, I came to acceptance.

Now, I don't wish to mislead you. It didn't happen quickly or in sequence. Acceptance is pernicious. Just as you believe you have made the ultimate adjustment, a new symptom arises, and you fall into the old cycle of denial, anger, and depression. Slowly, I found that the grieving times were growing shorter and my ability to accept things easier—that I would be just as happy doing less and enjoying it more. I began to record my moods through this process. I wrote lengthy e-mails to my distant friends and reread them every once in a while. I saw the pattern, and gradually I came to accept—and, yes, even *like*—having time to savor the moment. As much as I had valued "busyness," I discovered it wasn't at all necessary for a happy life.

Acceptance, I found, was empowering. Gradually, I began to notice more. Every time I had a good day, everything, from the rising sun to the smiles on faces around me, had meaning. I found that acceptance meant seeing myself as someone who, along with my personal qualities and idiosyncrasies, was also a person with Sjögren's syndrome. I was not, as I had described myself earlier, my disease! Acceptance meant allowing myself to rest when I was tired, find pleasure in simpler activities, and choose to do only what my body allowed.

It certainly hasn't been easy. I am equally certain that there are many rough patches ahead. When I struggled with the early diagnosis there was never enough information. Dr. Carteron was a wellspring of information, always encouraging, assuring me that I would survive. Being an ornery cuss, I wanted to research the condition without constantly running back to her for reassurance. I wanted control. What I learned instead was that we are a team and that to keep up my side of the effort, I must know when I can do something to help and when I cannot. I studied everything I could find about Sjögren's syndrome. Gradually, with Dr. Carteron's tutelage, I began to understand the disease and the efficacy of teamwork.

And so the idea for this book was born. I had learned so much, I hoped it would be useful to others. I had learned about "cutting edge" techniques that might help others and had the good fortune to work with a doctor for whom "new" (and sometimes "old") meant "worth trying." I will always be grateful to her.

While *A Body Out of Balance* is many things, it cannot be all things to all patients. That is because each of us is unique and will present symptoms different from those of another. We hope this book provides the road map to the territory of Sjögren's syndrome. The directions must come from the teamwork of the informed patient and a caring doctor. We sincerely hope to provide guidance and inspiration.

I couldn't have done this without the support of the members of the East Bay Support Group of the Sjögren's Syndrome Foundation. To them, I offer my thanks, prayers for good quality of health, and joy in their daily lives.

—RUTH FREMES, M.A.
Berkeley, California
January 2003

Introduction
by Nancy Carteron, M.D., the Doctor

THERE ARE DAYS WHEN I FEEL LIKE A MEDICAL Sherlock Holmes. Like Holmes, my work as a rheumatologist is based on detection. Daily I am presented with mysterious unconnected elusive symptoms which when considered along with scientific knowledge can eventually lead us to a diagnosis. With that diagnosis we can move to a treatment and ultimately to a patient's relief. The opportunity to help patients in this way is challenging, and truthfully, very rewarding. It is exciting to help solve a puzzle that has so disrupted a person's life. It can be a laborious process and one that takes many years to accomplish, but with patience and partnership between doctor and patient, it is possible.

In my experience, patients with autoimmune diseases have an even more difficult path than those with acute diseases. Autoimmune diseases are variable, chronic, and often begin when the patient is quite young and so last a lifetime. Further confounding the process is our health-care system, which focuses on the "cure" of an illness rather than its management. I have often heard patients lament that they would rather have a broken leg than autoimmunity. A leg gets attention and can be "fixed" whereas autoimmune diseases have attracted little support and much less interest within the medical community. It takes patience, detective work, and research, but answers can be found and treatment and healing plans can be designed, and better health—even remissions—are possible. I have seen this consistently in my practice. As you read Ruth Fremes's Introduction, it should become clear just how satisfying this work is to a physician. To help those who have suffered for so long with undiagnosed symptoms brings great rewards. In the same way, I am grateful for the opportunity to collaborate with her in writing this book.

We have tried to make Sjögren's syndrome accessible to you; we hope we have succeeded. If so, and if it helps in your journey to wellness, I am grateful. I believe strongly in these healing strategies and hope that they will assist you in your search for a peaceful and healthy quality of life.

I would also like to thank Drs. Phil Tumulty and Mary Betty Stevens, early mentors at Johns Hopkins Medicine, who introduced me to the world of patients with autoimmune diseases.

—NANCY CARTERON, M.D., FACR
California Pacific Medical Center
San Francisco, California
January 2003

What You Can Expect from This Book

WHATEVER YOUR RELATIONSHIP WITH SJÖGREN'S syndrome (SjS) today, you can expect this book to provide information and support in your search for a pleasant quality of life.

We will begin with explanations of autoimmune diseases and of SjS so that you can begin to understand what is happening in your body. Because it can affect every gland and organ in the body, we will take you on a body tour, explaining as we go how the disorder can invade different tissues and what to expect when it does. If you need help organizing your thoughts before you see your doctor, we have a section on what to take with you to that first appointment, what to expect, and how to get the most from the ongoing relationship with your doctor. In the second section, we will offer help for the pain and inconveniences that accompany the disorder by providing suggestions and explanations of both traditional prescription medicines and simpler, more homespun ones. In some cases, it is essential to use the high-powered drugs; in others, a milder palliative will do. In every case, nutrition plays a major part in helping you feel well. Our chapters on nutrition and stress management include the very latest information available on autoimmunity and lifestyle changes.

It's said that knowledge is power. Never before has that power been more necessary. The days of the dependent patient are over. An informed patient can do a lot to enhance the care that a good physician provides.

Knowledge brings independence, and independence can lead to partnership.

The aim of this book is to improve your quality of life. We hope to guide you through the search for information, help you with understanding, and empower you to become an informed partner with your physicians in the treatment process. We will offer new and effective ways to manage the symptoms and discuss how to overcome the emotional toll that comes from having to cope with a chronic disease.

When you do not know what your symptoms mean, it is devastating. When you learn what the symptoms mean, it is life-giving.

I get up.
I walk. . . .
I fall down.
Meanwhile, I keep dancing.

—HILLEL

A Body
Out of Balance

1

Understanding Sjögren's Syndrome

IF YOU'RE LEAFING THROUGH THIS BOOK FOR THE first time, chances are good that the diagnosis of Sjögren's syndrome (SjS) is new to you. Perhaps you've had a few persistent symptoms that you couldn't explain but that your doctor has suggested could be autoimmunity, specifically something called Sjögren's syndrome. Or you have been experiencing dry eyes and dry mouth and your doctor or dentist suggested a cause—Sjögren's syndrome. Or maybe you've been searching the Internet for an explanation of your symptoms, and SjS seems to fit the bill.

> My eyes were the least of my worries until I was diagnosed and realized that my eyes were causing me a problem, small though it was. I am fortunate in that respect. My mouth was very dry and I thought I was thirsty, and had anyone asked me if I was "dry," I would have answered "no." If I had seen a brochure lying around that talked about dryness symptoms, I would have ignored it. My symptoms were multiple, and nobody put it all together. I had pain and swelling in my hand, arm, and elbow; suffered with chronic sinus problems; depression; thirst; persistent dry cough; and intermittent pain throughout the body. I had never heard of Sjögren's syndrome. Once I received the diagnosis, I had a thousand questions.
>
> —Charlotte

Her confusion is understandable. It may be comforting to have a diagnosis after suffering with the symptoms for so long, but after a time, questions must come up—what is this syndrome? And what does it mean in my life?

Defining Sjögren's Syndrome

It was a Swedish ophthalmologist, Henrik Sjögren (pronounced SHOW-gren), who, along with his ophthalmologist wife, observed that a large number of his patients with chronic arthritis were also suffering with dry eyes and dry mouth. He described nineteen patients, all female, between the ages of twenty-nine and seventy-two, who had these complaints. Of the nineteen, thirteen also had chronic arthritis. In a few of those with arthritis, he also found microscopic features of chronic inflammation in the inflamed arthritic tissues. That was in 1933. A decade later the concept of autoimmune disorders emerged as well as a better understanding of SjS.

All autoimmune disorders—some localized, some systemic—are similar in their mechanisms. They all exhibit changes of chronic inflammation in tissues with an absence of any obvious chronic infection. The American Autoimmune Related Diseases Association (AARDA) reports that one in five Americans, or 20 percent of the population, has an autoimmune disease. Sjögren's syndrome (SjS), which is now recognized as one of the most common but often undiagnosed of the fifty-six known autoimmune diseases, is estimated to affect 4 million people in the United States alone. SjS is a chronic autoimmune and inflammatory disorder in which the body's immune system reacts against itself, primarily destroying the exocrine or mucous-secreting glands as though they were foreign bodies.

What Is Autoimmunity?

The fifty-six known autoimmune disorders are a large and highly variable group, but they are all the consequence of a loss of balance in the normal immune system. In a normally functioning immune system, immune cells are summoned into action to produce antibodies to counter *antigens* (infectious agents) in order to destroy them, as in, let's say, influenza. As long as the antigen is there, antibodies are produced, often causing inflammation. But influenza has an end. The body's antibodies, given time and assistance from proteins called *complements,* will destroy the virus or antigen. The resulting debris is then neatly removed from the body. But in the case of autoimmune disorders, it is impossible to destroy the antigen; it's a part of us.

Autoimmunity is similar to being allergic to yourself because your body actually makes antibodies that attack its own tissues. In other words, your body comes under "friendly fire" as your immune system cells attack "self" tissue. Since our body's mechanism of tolerance to "self" tissue has been broken, the body is in a constant state of conflict.

WHAT CAUSES AUTOIMMUNITY?

Autoimmunity is *not* directly caused by an infectious agent such as hepatitis C, Epstein-Barr, HIV, parvirus B19, or retroviruses, although they and others have been implicated in "triggering" its development. Viruses may trigger the process, but it is the immune system that mounts the attack and fuels the ongoing battle.

Current thinking about the cause of autoimmunity suggests that there is an interplay of triggering agents such as genetics, gender differences, and the unique characteristics of each person, at work. It is postulated that a triggering agent such as a virus, possibly a retrovirus, causes a series of events in a predisposed person that result in SjS. A particularly toxic flu could cause a very high fever that leads to a feeling of chronic ill health, which could be the beginning of autoimmunity. The initial flu virus could be the first pull of the trigger for the disease process, but it is not the weapon of battle; that was the immune system.

Many possible causes of autoimmunity are being investigated but have yet to be proven. Contributing to the process, but again not the single cause, are hormonal factors. Because so many sufferers are women, researchers are investigating the hormonal component of this complex process. Other studies focus on the residual fetal cells found in SjS patients. In all likelihood, some of us are more likely to develop autoimmune diseases because of our genetic profile. Then again, some people believe that the stresses of our everyday life may make us more susceptible. Family strife, job insecurities, and frustrations of any kind, if steady and intense enough, will change a person's neuroendocrine and hormonal profile in a way that allows other factors to take over, with the outcome a possible autoimmune disorder.

This growing knowledge base, while still very far from complete, is bringing us closer to discovering how SjS develops. Although exciting research is unfolding almost daily, until we understand the mechanism behind autoimmunity more completely, we will be forced to treat the symptoms of the disorder rather than its cause, for which there is not yet a one-time systemic cure or vaccine. There is intense ongoing research into the details of why and how many factors are exerting their effect in autoimmune diseases. Results of this research will likely translate into a better understanding of the process, earlier diagnosis, and better therapies for patients. Already there are some systemic and specific medications that

---

The Doctor's Observations

My experience of working with patients over the past twenty years has led me to conclude (as others have) that autoimmune diseases occur on a continuum. First, there will be a "stress event," often an infectious agent, like the "flu" or other virus, but just as likely an environmental stressor, such as a drug, followed by an abnormally long inflammatory response. For reasons we do not fully understand, the body's usual check-and-balance functions are not effective, and autoimmunity occurs. In severe cases it develops into a full-blown autoimmune disorder.

Even when in remission, once autoimmunity has been triggered, flare-ups of symptoms occur much more easily. Autoimmunity can be characterized as having an evolving, relapsing, and remitting course. This variability in occurrence of symptoms makes autoimmunity difficult to diagnose. Often, patients make an appointment for diagnosis when in a "flare," only to have the symptoms subside once they are ready for testing. But eventually, the disorder will recur, giving physicians the opportunity to intervene, reestablish balance, prevent disease progression, and modulate the severity of "flares." The challenging nature of the diagnosis and treatment of autoimmunity demands a good relationship between doctor and patient. Patients need to accurately inform the doctor of the changes in symptoms as they occur, giving the physician the chance to help in the progression of the disorder.

As a medical community, we do not fully understand how to return balance to the immune system once it has been affected. We can help induce remissions and instruct patients on how to manage the symptoms, but we cannot correct the problem—yet!

—Nancy Carteron, M.D.

were not in the pharmacies five years ago. With more enlightening research, the number of suffering patients will be much reduced in the near future.

How Does the Immune System Work?

Every cell in the body has a protective wall around it that resists invaders. Skin and the mucous membranes that exist in every body cavity and tract are designed to repel microbes and foreign substances. Mucous secretions, including saliva, tears, earwax, fuming acidic gastric juices, and sweat, are admirably suited to keep out invading microorganisms. There are natural body processes, such as coughing, sneezing, vomiting, fever, diarrhea, and sweating, that aid this process. In addition to these elaborate protective mechanisms, there is a highly sophisticated immune system designed to protect the body from more deliberate microbial and allergic invasions.

The immune system is our body's protection against the multitude of microbes, or living cells, that co-inhabit our bodies for better and for worse. Some of these microbes, especially those in the digestive system, produce vitamins that we use each day, facilitate the digestion and absorption of nutrients, and aid in the excretion of toxic substances. But many of these microorganisms can become virulent if they reach a vital organ such as the liver or kidneys, where they have the potential to change the normal functions of the cells in these organs, which in turn can cause a wide variety of diseases, some fatal. We depend totally on our immune systems to prevent *pathogenic* (disease-causing) microbes from becoming dangerous and harmful.

The immune system is also a powerful defender against other foreign substances and molecules, such as allergens, fungi, and parasites. The immune system protects our bodies from thousands of assaults each day, leaving us unaware we are ever at risk.

THE LYMPHATIC SYSTEM

While the body's immune response involves many parts of the body, central command is in the lymphatic system. Operating similarly to the circulatory system and its blood vessels, the lymphatic system circulates the *lymph* (fluid-containing white blood cells) through capillaries and vessels throughout the body. This system meets to form two lymphatic ducts, which join two large blood veins in the shoulder area.

There are a number of lymphatic organs or glands essential to the immune response of the body. These are the lymph nodes, situated throughout the lymphatic system; the thymus gland, behind the sternum; the spleen, in the upper left side of the abdominal cavity; and the tonsils, which are arranged in a ring at the junction of the nasal and oral cavities. The key element of successful immune responses is the system's ability to distinguish what's "us" and what's "not us"—between cells and molecules that are native and those that are foreign.

White Blood Cells

The basic functions of the lymphatic system are performed by white blood cells, or *leukocytes.* Twenty-five percent of white blood cells are a type of cell called *lymphocytes,* which occur in several forms: natural killer cells, macrophages (phagocytic cells), T cells, and B cells. Lymphocytes are formed in the bone marrow and thymus, and are modified into various forms in different parts of the lymphatic system to perform specific tasks.

The natural killer cells attack abnormal body cells that are virus-infected or tumor cells. Natural killer cells play a vital role in slowing and eliminating viruses and the spread of tumors by rupturing such cells and summoning phagocytes to destroy them. Phagocytic cells engulf and destroy undesirable substances or microorganisms, mobilizing immune cells and *lysosomes* (particles that contain enzymes capable of destroying foreign organisms). Once the battle is over, phagocytic cells help clear the dead cells and debris. The phagocytes die in battle and, along with the annihilated invaders, may accumulate at the site of the infection and form what's commonly regarded as pus.

The T cells are so called because they are lymphocytes that are formed in the bone marrow and then mature in the thymus gland—T for thymus. T cells are particularly involved in cell-mediated immunity, immunity that occurs when cells actually destroy the foreign agent. They are also utilized against multicellular parasites, cells infected with bacteria or viruses, and organ and tissue transplants. They act in part by releasing special proteins called *lymphokines,* which help coordinate the activities of the T cells, the B cells, and the macrophages.

B cells, which are produced and mature in the bone marrow, are involved in antibody-mediated immunity. B cells produce antibodies, relatively large water-soluble protein molecules that circulate readily in blood, lymph, and tissue fluids. Examples of antibodies are immunoglobulins such as IgG and IgM. These antibodies react with specific foreign molecules, called *antigens,* which are found on or in invading bacteria, toxins, viruses, or other molecules.

THE IMMUNE REACTION

The body's immune response is a systematic, effective process that involves the lymphatic, circulatory, and endocrine systems. It's swift and often specific. It holds information for years, even over a lifetime, in what is called *immune memory.* So, a case of measles that has been fought successfully will confer on you a lifelong immunity against that disease. In normal immune function, lymphocytes increase in number in response to infection or foreign bodies. Often, physicians measure white blood cell count in order to assess the strength or weakness of the immune system.

Antigens

The immune-system response begins with antigens. Most antigens are large protein molecules, although some are *polysaccharides* (carbohydrates in nature). Antigens serve as recognition markers for the T and B cells and indicate on the surface of a cell if it is "self" or "nonself." The self-antigens designate those cells that are particular to an individual; the nonself antigens designate foreign cells, such as bacteria, fungi, parasites, pollen grains, or mold spores. Their presence on foreign cells provokes the production of antibodies by the B cells and the attack by the T cells. The name *antigen* is actually derived from the phrase "antibody-generating molecule."

Antigens are water soluble and may be in circulation on their own or in cluster with other molecules in the blood, the lymph, or extracellular fluid. Antigens have the potential to invoke several types of immune responses in the body. Antigens may imbed themselves on the surface of cells but remain partially exposed, making them recognizable to T cells, thereby initiating an immune response. Sometimes phagocytes engulf antigens and present small fragments to the T cells as a means of augmenting the immune response. In other instances, phagocytes may destroy antigens directly.

T-Cell Response

As noted above, T cells are responsible for the cell-mediated immune response. After coming into contact with a nonself antigen, T cells can also store information necessary to identify the antigen in their surface receptors. They then form memory T cells and lie dormant so they can attack these antigens with precision and specificity if they show up again in the future.

After maturing in the thymus, T cells are transformed into one of two forms carrying either CD-4 or CD-8 protein characteristics. The CD-4 T cells act by quickly cloning themselves to produce large quantities of various interleukins, which stimulate the action of B cells, CD-8 T cells, and natural killer cells. Together, these cells mount a swift, precise attack aimed at the cells that hold the nonself antigen in question. Because CD-4 T cells regulate all of these functions, they are often referred to as "helper" T cells.

The CD-8 T cells have the capacity to recognize infected cells or tumor cells. In order to destroy the diseased cells, they clone themselves to form a critical mass of cytotoxic T cells, which produce *perforins* or a similar toxic substance to puncture the membranes of infected cells and lymphotoxins to fragment the DNA of invading cells.

There is some experimental evidence that there may exist a type of T cell, referred to as a *suppressor T cell*, that terminates the immune response once the battle is won and the antigen is no longer there.

B-Cell Response

The B cell is responsible for antibody-mediated immunity, in an analogous and complementary way to the cell-mediated response of the T cells. Once mature, the B cells move into the bloodstream to reside in the lymphatic system. The antibodies they produce circulate freely throughout the blood and the extracellular fluid.

The B cells themselves carry receptors that target and bind with specific antigens. This binding activates B cells to clone themselves in order to outnumber and kill the enemy—the antigen-carrying nonself cells. As with the T cells, some of the B cells can lie dormant, holding immune memory for future defenses. There is also some evidence that once the enemy is destroyed, suppressor T cells may step in to put an end to the B cell fire.

Immune Response in SjS

Autoimmune disorders like SjS represent a failure of the T and B cells to distinguish between the self and the nonself antigens: The immune system launches an attack against the body's own tissues. There is a group of genes, known as *human leukocyte antigens* (HLA), that control the ability of the T and B cell to respond to self and nonself antigens. We suspect that the misguided response of the immune system to self antigens lies in the HLA complex. There may also be the added complication of the inability of the suppressor T cells to step in to stop this harmful misguided attack on the self cells.

One of the ways in which T cells influence immune function is through production of molecules called *cytokines*. Experimental studies are currently focusing on two of the most important pro-inflammatory cytokines: tumor necrosis factor alpha (TNF alpha) and interleukin-1 (IL-1). These have been found to be key promoters of inflammation in the autoimmune disorder rheumatoid arthritis, and data support the role of these cytokines in SjS as well.

There is an additional housekeeping task our bodies perform. All cells have a predetermined life span, and when they die, they are cleared from the body in a process called *apoptosis*, which does not induce an inflammatory reaction. In autoimmune disorders, apoptosis may malfunction, causing cells to accumulate in the body. This cell buildup, in part, is responsible for *lymphoma* (cancer of the lymphocytes). Lymphoma or pseudolymphoma (not quite lymphoma) may occur in SjS.

New research is pointing to another lymphocyte intracellular signaling pathway, called the *toll-like receptor-signaling pathway*, as having a role in developing autoimmunity. This particular pathway becomes involved when the immune cells see bacterial fragments, and may be the key to understanding how autoimmune diseases are connected to infectious organisms.

Understanding Sjögren's Syndrome

Now how does autoimmunity translate into a disease in a given individual? Generally, autoimmune diseases can be divided into two categories: those where the immune system attacks multiple organs and those where it attacks a single organ. For example, *systemic lupus erythematosus* (SLE or lupus) can attack multiple organs. The attack is mounted toward the *nucleosome* (DNA plus histone [protein] clumps) in cells. Since this complex is present in almost all cells that make up specific organs, the disease can affect any organ in the body. This causes a multitude of varying symptoms from joint pain to mouth sores. In contrast, Hashimoto's thyroiditis results from an attack on a single organ, the thyroid, and rheumatoid arthritis occurs when the *synovium* (joint-lining tissue) is attacked.

Although many parts of our bodies can be affected by SjS—lungs, brain, nerves, joints, kidneys, and liver, to name a few—in the majority of cases, the autoimmune response is confined to the lacrimal (tear) and salivary (mouth) glands. In this way, SjS should be quickly diagnosed when the primary symptoms are dry eyes and mouth. SjS may range in severity from a mild inconvenience to serious and worrisome problems. Although at times you can feel deathly ill or frustratingly disabled, it is rare to have any of these symptoms develop into life-threatening conditions. Very rarely, lymphocytes of the immune system transform into cancer cells and lymphoma develops, but this occurs over years and is predated by a condition known as pseudolymphoma. If this is detected early, it can usually be cured or effectively managed.

Why Me?

The most natural response to a diagnosis of Sjögren's syndrome is to wonder "why me?" What did I do (or not do) to bring on this confounding disorder? Is it in my genes? What is the prognosis?

Well, the answers aren't simple. Medical science acknowledges that you may have gotten the syndrome for reasons as yet undiscovered. The

---

I am twenty-four and have just been diagnosed with SjS after going through many tests. I was deeply fatigued, falling asleep at inappropriate times, often in front of the computer at work. My joints hurt, mostly in the mornings, and I wondered if it could all be psychological. Now I wonder whether it is usual for someone so young to get this disease. And I wonder what will happen as I get older. I wonder what is happening in my body. And why did *I* get it?

—Debbie

cause of SjS is still under investigation, but there are many things that may indicate an increased risk. Anyone can get SjS; it affects all ages and all races. SjS is more common in women than in men; in fact, nine out of ten people who get SjS are women. Why this is has not been fully explained, but it is widely accepted that the important influence of sex hormones on immunoregulation and autoimmunity is a key factor. SjS is more likely to develop in the perimenopausal years. The mean age at diagnosis is fifty years, but this age may not be entirely accurate since SjS is difficult to diagnose and often patients put off seeking medical counsel.

There are actually two peak ages of onset. A younger group of patients (ages twenty to forty years) frequently experiences the onset of dry eyes and systemic manifestations similar to those of patients with lupus (SLE) and are often classified as having lupus with secondary SjS. In a second group of patients, SjS onset doesn't occur until age sixty or older and generally involves fewer systemic manifestations. This older group closely overlaps the population of those diagnosed with lupus at an older age, and its members are also often diagnosed as having lupus with secondary SjS. In addition, secondary SjS can occur in children as part of the spectrum of juvenile rheumatoid arthritis.

You may be more likely to develop SjS if you already have another autoimmune disorder such as rheumatoid arthritis, lupus, scleroderma, polymyositis, dermatomyositis, systemic vasculitis, celiac disease, primary biliary cirrhosis, chronic active hepatitis, idiopathic Addison's disease, or insulin-dependent diabetes.

You could be at higher risk if you carry certain genes, termed *histocompatibility antigens* (HLA), thus giving you a genetic predisposition.

Primary Sjögren's Syndrome
Definite dry eyes
Definite dry mouth
Absence of any other cause (such as rheumatoid arthritis)

Secondary Sjögren's Syndrome
Dry eyes and/or mouth in association with an autoimmune disorder, most commonly lupus (SLE) and rheumatoid arthritis

Those who have the HLA-B8 and DR3 phenotype (the physical manifestation of a particular gene) are more likely to get primary SjS. Interestingly, this association is not found in those with secondary SjS.

As for doing something to bring on SjS, the doctor's answer is a definite "no!" You did not do anything to deserve this disorder. You have no control over whether you are born female, have certain genes, have red or brown hair, or caught a virus that may have triggered your system to react in this way.

The good news is that for the most part you can gain control over SjS. You can learn about it, study your body's reactions to the stresses and strains of life, help control the symptoms, and even halt the progression. At times, the symptoms become overwhelming, and at other times, they cause only a minor irritation. The more you learn about the disease, the symptoms, and the signs, the more likely you are to have a comfortable life.

A patient is said to have either primary or secondary SjS depending upon the presence or absence of another autoimmune disorder. If someone

The Symptoms and Signs of Sjögren's Syndrome		
SYMPTOMS		
Eyes	**Mouth**	**Other**
Chronic feeling of grittiness like sand or grain in the eye	Dry mouth	Fatigue
Burning sensation	Difficulty chewing and swallowing dry foods such as dry crackers	Malaise or depression
Itching	Burning or sore mouth	Sleep disturbance; frequent awakening due to dryness
Sticky eyelids after sleep	Frequent dental fillings	Intermittent joint pain
Few tears or decreased tearing	Abnormal taste	Muscle pain
Oily feeling at the corner of the eyes	Hoarseness	Frequent infections (bronchitis or sinusitis)
Light sensitivity; need to squint	Trouble wearing dentures	Vaginal dryness and yeast infections
Redness	Tender gums	Skin dryness
Filmy sensation affecting vision	Dry, sticky feeling in the mouth	Constipation
Short distance vision; problems while reading, doing computer work, sewing, etc.	Excessive thirst	Nausea, abdominal pain, and tenderness
	Sensitive to spicy or acidic foods	Inflammatory skin rashes

WHAT YOUR DOCTOR LOOKS FOR

Eyes	Mouth	Other
Positive Schirmer's test	Multiple areas of decay	Raynaud's disease
Low tear breakup time when fluoresein is instilled into tear film	Cracked teeth	Inflammatory skin rashes indicating vasculitis
Positive rose bengal score	Problems with dental crowns	Low white blood cell count
Mucus and debris stuck on the eye surface as seen by biomicroscopy	Enlargement of the salivary gland, submandibular and/or parotid	Anemia
Perforation of the cornea that can occur with severe dry eye when a corneal ulcer becomes infected	Decreased salivary pool beneath the tongue	Dry, cracked lips
	Thick, whitish saliva expressed from salivary gland ducts	
	Wooden tongue depressor adheres to the tongue	
	Oral candida as seen in a red, fissured tongue	
	Redness and cracking at the corners of the mouth	
	Lipstick on the teeth	
	Salivary gland biopsy showing focal lymphocyte infiltrates	

has rheumatoid arthritis and dry eye/dry mouth syndrome, they are said to have rheumatoid arthritis with secondary SjS.

FLARES

Remember the rhyme about the little girl with the curl on her forehead? When she was good, she was very, very good, but when she was bad, she was HORRID? Living with her would be a bit like living with SjS. When it's awful, we forget that it will ever be good again. But it will be; what goes up the teeter-totter must come down. You are simply living a "flare."

While there is little talk in the scientific literature of "flares" in SjS, clinical experience would argue that they are a common characteristic of the disease. A flare is a significant increase in intensity, frequency, and number of symptoms. Like a smoldering fire that erupts when someone adds lighter fluid, a flare describes an intensification of symptoms. These symptoms can be a resurgence either of old symptoms or of a constellation of symptoms that is unique to the patient. New symptoms can also develop over time. Sometimes arthritis symptoms will increase after an infection, or the dry eyes or dry mouth will worsen for a time after a period of stress. We can only hypothesize about the reasons for this.

Since the primary problem contributing to SjS seems to be immune deregulation, patients must be very conscious of any added strain on the body. Anything that will stimulate our immune system to act, such as an infection or added stress, could cause the immune system to remain on "alert" unnecessarily. It will remain vigilant even after the infection or stress has gone, thus bringing about a flare of symptoms. For example, chronic allergies can make you more susceptible to sinus infection. So check those allergies! Keep the nasal passages clear with daily saline rinses. And after a stressful event, it's best to be alert; allow extra time to heal.

How Is Sjögren's Syndrome Diagnosed?

Each diagnosis can be hard to determine, especially in the earlier, milder stage. Complaints of dry mouth and dry eye are common and can be caused by pharmaceuticals as well as other medical conditions. Oftentimes, the first hints of SjS are picked up by a dentist who wonders at the large number of cavities in a patient's mouth, or by an ophthalmologist who notices excessively dry eyes. It isn't often that we, as patients, can recognize and assemble a picture that would lead to a comprehensive diagnosis, and our family physicians, burdened by managed-care requirements, often don't have the time. Nevertheless, once there's a hint of a possibility of SjS, the patient should have a complete work-up.

The person most qualified to diagnose and treat your condition is a rheumatologist, preferably one for whom you have a recommendation from either a patient or another doctor. A rheumatologist is a subspecialist who has two or more years of additional training. Recommendations for qualified rheumatologists can be located through the American College of Rheumatology or local Arthritis Foundation organizations.

This consulting specialist will take a complete history, perform an examination, order and assess the blood and other tests, decide whether you fit the picture for SjS, and then refer you to specialists such as eye and mouth physicians for your immediate care. It is necessary to establish a good working relationship with your rheumatologist as it is he or she who will collaborate with you to make sure that you maintain an optimal quality of life. SjS is not, in most cases, life-threatening. It is a chronic condition that requires attention from both physician and patient over a lifetime.

What Is the Prognosis When the Diagnosis Is SjS?

The prognosis with regard to major problems is very good. Usually patients will be bothered by the symptoms related to the decrease and defective quality of the secretions from the exocrine glands. Occasionally, the rapid increase of lymphocytes in the exocrine glands of the respiratory tract, vagina, pancreas, and bladder may result in chronic or frequent symptoms related to those organs such as cough, vaginal dryness, abdominal pain, or urinary tract infections. Arthritis can develop, but it is not aggressive or destructive like rheumatoid arthritis. Mild nervous-system symptoms can occur such as depression, tingling, or numbness, and the kidneys can be affected. Very rarely the lungs can become inflamed and scarring can occur. Sometimes the body makes too much of certain immunoglobulins, which cause specific symptoms such as fatigue and joint pain.

Lymphomas can develop in up to 9 percent of SjS patients. Most of these lymphomas are B-cell lymphomas. The biopsy diagnosis is usually non-Hodgkin's lymphoma or MALToma. But, as we said earlier, this type of lymphoma is usually slow to develop and very responsive to therapy.

Physicians tend to focus on the benign nature of SjS while patients experience the often intense discomfort of its symptoms. This difference in perspective is understandable; physicians see diseases that are far deadlier than SjS while a patient is only aware of the severity of the symptoms she or he is suffering. An empathetic doctor and an informed patient will produce the most optimal and supportive care.

How Can I Feel Better?

SjS cannot be cured—yet. We're close, but as yet no treatment has been found to replace the glandular secretions that are symptomatic of SjS. Researchers are working on pinpointing the origins of the disorder and concomitantly on how to avoid its onset, but so far our treatment options are aimed at symptom relief and prevention of tissue damage.

The goals of treatment are twofold: to provide relief from the symptoms and to reduce the risk of long-term damage. There are several approaches, depending upon the severity of the condition at the time. There are topical additions to help lubricate eyes and mouth, such as artificial tears and mouth lubricants. Fortunately for us, the pharmaceutical manufacturers who prepare remedies for dry eyes, mouth, and other symptoms have found it to be in their financial interest to improve their products. Consequently, the eye moisteners and mouth gels that are on the market today are far superior to those of the past, and we believe they can only get better. Closing the tear drains (punctal occlusion) can help dry eyes in some people. Nonsteroidal anti-inflammatory drugs (NSAIDs), like ibuprofen, have improved in recent years. They are recommended to reduce the swelling of enlarged and inflamed glands and to relieve joint and muscle pain. In some cases, a physician will prescribe systemic medicines, such as hydroxychloroquine or corticosteroids to help reduce inflammation, or pilocarpine or cevimiline to increase glandular secretions, and in troubling cases, immunosuppressive drugs like methotrexate will be used. But in general, the symptoms are treated with simple remedies.

Along with the battery of pharmaceutical remedies come recommendations for lifestyle changes that will greatly help improve the symptoms. Dietary changes such as the ones we explain in Chapter 11 and stress-reduction techniques such as those we discuss in Chapter 12 will have a surprising impact on how you feel each day.

For further information, please see Resources, page 165.

CHAPTER 2

Discovering a Diagnosis

THE FIRST MEETING OF DOCTOR AND PATIENT IS
critical. The patient has eagerly waited to tell her story to a caring, knowledgeable, and helpful listener with the capacity to heal; the doctor will be listening like a detective for clues as the story unfolds. From the information the patient provides, the doctor will get a sense of the possible source of her patient's distress. For the best diagnosis, the patient will need to tell her story clearly and chronologically since she last felt well, using the "Personal Health History" (see page 39) as a guide. The doctor will listen for evidence that, when pieced together, will form a possible explanation or hypothesis for the symptoms.

To illustrate how one patient found a diagnosis and treatment of Sjögren's syndrome, we will use the case study of a patient named Alice. This chapter will take you step by step through the diagnosis process and illustrate how Alice worked with her doctor to find a treatment path. Each SjS patient's symptoms and experiences are unique. But Alice is a typical example of an SjS patient with extraglandular involvement—she experiences symptoms beyond dry eyes and mouth, joint pain, and fatigue.

There are four components to a thoughtful, careful consultation: (1) time, (2) past history of illness, (3) specialist physical examination, and (4) tests. Doctors often need additional time for medical literature research and for consultation with subspecialty colleagues knowledgeable in autoimmunity.

Alice

Alice came to the doctor complaining of pain, fatigue, and dryness. She had suffered for years and felt defeated by the medical runaround that had taken her from doctor to doctor. It began about six years ago, when she was in her mid-fifties. She was an avid skier who spent every spare minute on the slopes. One day, while on a family holiday, she noticed her arms and shoulders were very painful to touch. She was unusually sore after skiing, but this pain was new and unusual for her. Soon after this, she began experiencing screaming pain in her legs when she climbed the stairs. Around the same time, she began feeling chronically fatigued. She found herself falling asleep in business meetings. She tried to explain that this wasn't ordinary fatigue; it was exhaustion unlike anything she had known. Her mouth was also so dry that she had to sip water constantly just to be able to speak, which interfered with her job as a mortgage broker.

Her doctor suggested that although he could see nothing definitive, her fatigue and pain could be caused by fibromyalgia. He also told her that her vaginal dryness and fatigue could also be hormone-related. To combat the dryness and fatigue, she began hormone replacement therapy, and to soothe her pain, she and her husband tried massage therapy. But her pain was too severe for massage therapy to work and too intense even for the physiotherapy her doctor suggested.

Alice's ailments persisted and were joined by new and even more troubling ones. She had nausea for no reason, headache where there was none before, and general distress in her stomach. The gastrointestinal specialist performed a gastric endoscopy and found stomach ulcers. He suggested they could probably be traced back to the over-the-counter pain and inflammation medication she had been taking regularly to relieve the joint stiffness.

Confused and frustrated, Alice fell into a slump. She could no longer put in a full working day. Increasingly, her husband was distant and absorbed in his own thoughts. Intercourse, which had always been pleasurable, had become painful, and she and her husband made love less and less. Her marriage was crumbling. Her illness seemed to have taken her life for ransom. She felt isolated and angry. It wasn't until six years after her first symptoms appeared that she experienced dry eyes and a slight change in her saliva flow and her family doctor sent her for a rheumatology consultation at a nearby teaching hospital.

Time

A first visit should be adequately paced, lasting about an hour with the specialist and additional time with the doctor's staff. A second hour is planned to avert any concerns the patient may have about medications, insurance, and the disorder itself. If there is not enough time for a relaxed interview, a patient may become flustered, and the doctor will elicit an incomplete history. If the history is very complicated or the patient unfocused, it may take several visits to compile a complete and accurate picture of her condition. It is very important that the patient be prepared and put at ease, and that the doctor allow enough time to gain a complete picture.

The amount of time allotted to this visit is a bellwether of both the physician's interest and expertise in these complicated conditions. Unfortunately, it may also be a function of the health-care environment. Most insurance companies underpay for diagnostic time, not acknowledging that complicated cases require extra time. This leaves the physician with one of two choices: require additional payment for the diagnostic process or give the patient too little time to do a complete assessment.

In order to ensure enough time for proper diagnoses, patients and physicians must be willing to put in an extra time commitment. Unfortunately, patients may have to pay for the extra time it takes to get a thorough examination out-of-pocket. A patient may also consider making a series of return visits in order to fully explore testing and diagnosis. This may be inconvenient, but insurance may pay for return visits. Patients should also consider themselves a partner with their doctor and always come to appointments in order to help and expedite the diagnoses process (see Chapter 3 for suggestions on how to prepare for visits to your physician).

Past History

This is the centerpiece of the interview, more important than tests or physical examination. The patient's story directs the investigative process. Alice tells a familiar story. She has been suffering for six years. Autoimmune and chronic inflammatory diseases often take a long time to coalesce around a comprehensive set of symptoms that suggests an appropriate diagnosis. Many things could have caused her symptoms. In addition, medications that have been used to treat allergy, blood pressure, or depression often contribute to further symptoms. Then again, the way she deals with stress also could be contributing to her symptoms. In some patients, menopause can cause similar symptoms. The doctor will ask targeted questions to rule out causes other than autoimmunity. The patient needs to be "patient," as the sorting process can take time.

Doctors will ask many questions when gathering a past history. They will attempt to flush out the information they need to form a hypothesis. The following are some questions a doctor would ask Alice upon her first consultation. With these questions, the physician is looking for specific clues that would warrant further investigative tests.

- *What were the first symptoms noticed?*

  For Alice, the first symptom of arm and shoulder pain in the shoulder girdle occurred on a ski trip but did not resolve as quickly as Alice would have expected. The degree of pain was out of proportion to the activity level, suggesting a more severe or "pathological" process. A possible hypothesis is inflammatory arthritis of the shoulder joint or surrounding tendons (rotator cuff), inflammation of the deltoid muscles (myositis), or a condition called *polymyalgia rheumatica* (PMR). On questioning, Alice reported that the shoulder pain never really left her, although at times it was less severe. Whatever your first symptom may have been, the doctor makes note of this and asks about other symptoms and what has helped the condition and what has not.

- *What are other symptoms?*

  Alice's severe fatigue mysteriously followed the shoulder girdle pain and tenderness. Then she noticed that her legs became painful when she walked. There was no history of trauma nor was there a "triggering event" that could account for it. Then she developed severe dry mouth (xerostomia), which interfered with her speech. Again, this arrived without explanation. She reports that carrying bottled water with her was necessary to remain hydrated enough to carry on a conversation, which is common among SjS patients.

- *Are there any other symptoms of autoimmunity such as a history of thyroiditis, a low white blood cell (WBC) or platelet count, or a family history of sarcoidosis (an autoimmune disorder characterized by small bumps on the lungs, spleen, liver, and skin)?*

  If you have had one autoimmune disorder, such as thyroiditis, you are at increased risk of developing another autoimmune disorder in the future. Often, patients with Sjögren's syndrome may have had decreased WBCs as a result of producing antibodies to their own WBCs, but the low count may come and go. If patients have also had decreased platelets and anemia (low red blood cells), this finding would be more compatible with another autoimmune disorder—lupus or autoimmune cytopenias.

- *What is your genetic family history?*

    Did any relative, no matter how distant, suffer with an autoimmune disorder like lupus, rheumatoid arthritis, psoriasis, thyroiditis, multiple sclerosis, or diabetes?

- *What medications do you take?*

    Chronic inflammation is suspected if you use NSAIDs (nonsteroidal anti-inflammatory drugs) often. In Alice's case it could also explain her stomach pain, as gastritis or peptic ulcer disease is brought on by steady ingestion of these medications. Antidepressants (SSRIs or tricyclics) could be one explanation for the dryness and could also be contributing to the severity of her symptoms. Allergy medications, too, can cause dryness.

- *What herbal remedies do you use?*

    Many teas and other caffeine drinks act as diuretics, which make dryness worse. Since most herbal remedies are not checked by the FDA for safety, efficacy, and interaction with prescription drugs or with each other, we can not exclude the possibility that they may worsen symptoms or cause others. During the diagnostic phase, your doctor may recommend that you keep medications and over-the-counter products to a minimum so as to observe your actual condition.

- *Do you have frequent infections?*

    This can be a significant clue to a diagnosis of SjS. In SjS the secretory glands are affected, and the protective antibodies of the mucosa (IgA) may be impaired, allowing infectious agents to enter the cells lining the mucosa of the sinuses and lungs more easily. Thus, new and recurrent upper respiratory infections (URIs), colds, and flus may be signs of SjS. If this is the case, the possibility also exists that an immunodeficiency disorder is present. If appropriate, immunology testing of your blood should be performed.

- *Do you often take antibiotics?*

    Some people may develop varying forms of immunodeficiency disorders when they do not have adequate protection against viral or bacterial agents; thus they may have an increasing frequency of infections that require frequent courses of antibiotics. If appropriate, immunology testing should be performed.

- *Did you experience a major infection, take new medication, or suffer major stressors before the problem began? If so, can you associate it with the onset of your symptoms?*

    All three of these can be triggers to autoimmunity. Infections in particular are noteworthy. Research is revealing that infectious agents continue to be major triggers of autoimmunity and chronic inflammation even after the immune system has effectively "killed" them.

- *Do you have a history of stomach ulcers?*

    It is not uncommon for those with autoimmune diseases to have stomach ulcers. Stomach ulcers can be caused by a bacteria, *H. pylori* (helicobacter). An immune response triggered by infections also could cause these symptoms or even cause further autoimmunity and infiltration of immune cells, usually lymphocytes, into the tissue lining the stomach and GI tract. Autoimmune patients ingest large numbers of nonsteroidal anti-inflammatory drugs to control their pain, and continued use of these drugs has been known to cause ulcers.

- *Describe your lifestyle today.*

    Talk about stress and how you handle it. How regular is your sleep? How adequate is your diet? Do you exercise, and if so, what is your routine? What supplements and alternative or complementary therapies and strategies have been successful for you?

General Physical Examination

Here today and gone tomorrow is the theme of autoimmune disease symptoms. Negative test findings aren't helpful, as symptoms may not be present the day of the test in spite of the fact that they were there yesterday or last month. A detailed history and review of systems is as necessary to the diagnostician as the physical examination. However, if autoimmune or inflammatory physical signs are present, they can be additional helpful clues.

SKIN

The doctor will begin by examining your skin, looking for evidence of red inflammatory rashes (tender nodules, hives), rash over the cheeks and bridge of the nose (malar rash), or clusters of small red blood vessels in the skin (telangiectasias); a lacy blood-vessel pattern often of the legs and arms (livedo reticularis); or mucous membrane (mouth, nose) ulcers. The nail beds (next to cuticle) of the hands and feet will also be examined as the doctor looks for any abnormal redness due to congestion of the capillaries (nail-bed erythema or blush). All of these symptoms would suggest a possible autoimmune disorder, possibly the inflammatory skin rashes or vasculitis that comes with SjS.

If the blood-vessel pattern on the skin exhibits a reddish blue mottling when exposed to cold, it could indicate an inflammatory or "spastic" reaction of the peripheral blood vessels. Your physician may also look for color changes of the hands and feet, which may range from red to white to blue (Raynaud's disease), which could indicate SjS. These symptoms are indicative of other diseases, so a positive physical finding does not assure an autoimmune diagnosis. For example, "splinter hemorrhages" on the digits (fingers or toes) can be a sign of small-vessel inflammation due to drugs, infections, or another rheumatic disease, or a sign of bacterial endocarditis (emboli from infection of the heart valve).

MOUTH

Your physician will examine your mouth, looking for the size of the salivary pool and moisture in the mucosa, and the condition of the tongue. A dry, cracked, "beefy" red tongue can be a sign of insufficient moisture or candida, a chronic yeast infection.

HAIR

Hair quality, quantity, and growth pattern will be checked by the physician. Thinning hair can be a sign of skin irregularities and an indicator of insufficient moisture getting to the scalp. This, along with other symptoms, can point to SjS.

GENERAL BODY EXAMINATION

The physician will test ligaments and tendons for pain due to inflammation. Feel for nodules on joints and check their location.

Diagnostic Tests

There are several diagnostic tools a doctor can use to determine SjS. Some can be performed by a general practitioner, and some will require a referral to a specialist. Below is a description of the tests commonly used to help diagnose SjS as well as the standard diagnostic criteria for the disease.

BLOOD TESTS

The most common blood tests associated with SjS look for SSA (Rho) and SSB (La) antibodies. Both of these antibodies are directed against a ribonuclear protein that is often present in cells of SjS patients. The presence of both SSA and SSB antibodies is highly suggestive of Sjögren's syndrome. The SSA antibody is also commonly seen in lupus and congenital heart block.

Antinuclear antibodies (ANAs) are autoantibodies that are directed against self DNA present in the nucleus of cells. The presence of ANAs in a blood test is a hallmark of autoimmunity. The rheumatoid factor (RF) is another autoantibody directed against self, usually found in the IgM and sometimes IgG or IgA class of immunoglobulins (protein antibodies involved in immunity). The presence of these antibodies in the blood can indicate rheumatoid arthritis, and they are often seen in SjS. The presence of monoclonal or oligoclonal antibodies may also suggest autoimmunity or immune-system malignancy.

Another test for SjS looks for a group of proteins called complements that react in a cascade, one activating the next, that help attack antigens. When certain classes of antibodies recognize and attach to antigens, a cascade is activated and levels of complement components C_3 and C_4 become lowered. When a blood test finds the levels of C_3 and C_4 are low, it could be an indication of autoimmunity.

EYE TESTS

Consider a referral to an ophthalmologist for complete testing of the eyes to check for dryness, the condition of the retina, or for clues of autoimmune or ischemic retinopathy. For information about eye tests such as the Schirmer's test and the rose bengal test, see Chapter 4.

SALIVARY FLOW MEASUREMENT

This is a measure of the rate of salivary production flow from the salivary glands in the mouth. Normal flow is greater than 1.5 ml in fifteen minutes.

PAROTID FLOW MEASUREMENT

This test is a measure of the rate of saliva production from the parotid gland, which is located inside the cheek, near the ear. Dye is placed in the duct to look for blockages and inflammation.

SALIVARY GLAND BIOPSY

To take a biopsy of the salivary gland, a doctor will inject local anesthesia into an area of your mouth in order to remove a small piece of tissue from a minor salivary gland (usually on the lower lip). A stitch will be required to mend the biopsy site. The site will remain numb for a while, and you may experience pain afterward due to the high concentration of pain fibers in the tissue. The biopsy will be examined by a pathologist for the presence of lymphocytes (white blood cells).

GALLIUM SCAN

To perform a gallium scan, a radioactive imaging material (radionuclide) is injected into a vein and images taken at various time intervals. As the radionuclide circulates, it will accumulate in inflamed tissue and will be visible during the scan. The tissue can then be biopsied for more specific information.

NERVE BIOPSY

If your physician notices neurological symptoms such as regional numbness or weakness during your physical examination, she will likely refer you to a neurologist for further testing. A biopsy of the skin along the affected nerve can detect small fiber neuropathy that cannot be found with other methods such as nerve-conduction studies.

GI Testing

Depending on how troubling your GI symptoms such as pain, burning, and acid taste in the mouth are, your physician may refer you to a gastroenterologist for an assessment of your possible ulcerative condition. The test, an upper endoscopy, is performed by placing a tube with a camera down the esophagus into the stomach to look for ulcers, and biopsies may be taken to exclude a chronic bacterial infection (*Helicobacter pylori*). Additional GI symptoms related to SjS may include lower abdominal pain, bloating, and severe constipation. A gastroenterologist may perform an abdominal CT (computed tomography) scan, colonoscopy, and motility testing to test for masses, diverticulitis, polyps, or slow colon muscle function.

Diagnostic Criteria

Presently there is no international agreement on diagnostic criteria for SjS. Until now, there have been three criteria in common use: the EEC, San Francisco, and San Diego. The San Francisco criteria require a minor salivary-gland biopsy, and the San Diego criteria require an autoantibody blood test. The most liberal set of criteria is that of the European Economic Community (EEC), which relies simply on symptoms as assessed by the patient and doctor. The EEC criteria reveal many more SjS sufferers than the San Francisco or San Diego criteria do.

For practical purposes, you can be diagnosed with SjS if you satisfy the revised international classification criteria:

Ocular symptoms: A positive response to at least one of the following questions:

- Have you had daily, persistent, troublesome dry eyes for more than three months?
- Do you have a recurrent sensation of sand or gravel in the eyes?
- Do you use tear substitutes more than three times a day?

Oral symptoms: A positive response to at least one of the following questions:

- Have you had a daily feeling of dry mouth for more than three months?

- Have you had recurrently or persistently swollen salivary/neck glands for more than three months as an adult?
- Do you frequently drink liquids to aid in swallowing dry foods?

Ocular signs: Objective evidence of ocular involvement defined as a positive result for at least one of the following two tests:

- Schirmer's test, performed without anesthesia (<5 mm in 5 minutes)
- Rose bengal score or other ocular dye score (>4 according to van Bijsterveld's scoring system)

Histopathology: In minor salivary glands (obtained through normal-appearing mucosa), focal lymphocytic sialoadenitis, evaluated by an expert histopathologist, with a focus score of >1, defined as a number of lympho-cytic foci that are adjacent to normal-appearing mucous acini and contain more than 50 lymphocytes per 4 mm of glandular tissue.

Salivary gland involvement: Objective evidence of salivary gland involvement defined by a positive result for at least one of the following diagnostic tests:

- Unstimulated whole salivary flow (<1.5 ml in 15 minutes)
- Parotid sialography, an X-ray test taken after an injection of dye into the ducts, to reveal the presence of dilated salivary ducts (in either a punctate, cavitary, or destructive pattern), without the evidence of obstructions in the major ducts.
- Salivary scintigraphy, an imaging scan performed after the injection of a radionuclide (see gallium scan above), showing delayed uptake, reduced concentration, and/or delayed excretion of the tracer (the radionuclide).

Blood Tests:
- A blood test revealing the presence in the serum of the antibodies SSA/Ro or SSB/La antigens, or both.

SjS seems simple enough to diagnose when a patient has dryness in the eyes or mouth and positive SSA and SSB antibodies, but when the symptoms are diffuse muscle aches, fatigue, and pain, usually a patient like Alice will be diagnosed with the syndrome only after abnormal tests and tissue biopsy return. Thus, it is extremely important that a complete set of tests be ordered, and in some cases that the patient be followed over time to collect sufficient data for an accurate diagnosis.

Physicians who've had experience with SjS often skirt the official criteria requirements and determine the diagnosis based on the patient having at least three of the following: dry mouth as observed objectively by the physician, dry eyes as observed objectively by the physician, autoimmunity as reflected by the blood tests, and, if thought to be necessary, confirmation through histologic (cellular) analysis of a sample of the salivary gland (salivary gland biopsy), remembering that all other possible diagnoses have been excluded.

It is possible to suffer from SjS and still have test readings in the normal range. In fact, many patients relate just that. But, as time goes on, test results change. A physician may suspect SjS with normal test results but have nothing objective to go on. She may even say something like "Well, your test results are normal, but I believe you are suffering from . . ." A patient with symptoms but otherwise normal readings would be wise to question the physician carefully about this possibility and what treatment protocol would be helpful to try for symptom relief. Thus, treatment options can be tried even if the diagnosis is presumptive or possible SjS. At the testing stage, when a patient suffers from numerous symptoms, no possibility should be overlooked in order to reach the most accurate diagnosis.

UNDERSTANDING DIAGNOSTICS

When the doctor sends you to a lab for blood tests, she is looking for an overall picture of your health as well as indicators of autoimmunity. When the results come back, the values are compared with the standard specific to that laboratory. There is a lack of uniformity in the units used to report test results both nationally and internationally. It is always a good idea to get copies of your results and to keep them in a folder or binder for comparison with your doctor over time. Because of the differences among the labs, it is important to compare them only to the reference range on the sheet, not with published values that may not apply to you.

A general finding of SjS is made from tests when the SSA (Rho) and SSB (La) antibodies are positive; these antibodies are most often but not always found with a positive ANA antibody. Rheumatoid factor and low white blood cell count (WBC) are also common in SjS. The tissue biopsy showing lymphocytic infiltration measured by a "focus score" is also diagnostic of the syndrome.

The Diagnosis

For Alice, the most likely diagnoses are: fibromyalgia, menopause, and an autoimmune or inflammatory process. The doctor will have checked that the primary-care physician has ruled out cancer or an obvious infectious process. If there is a question of a cancer process that may have gone undetected, a referral will be made to an oncology specialist for a complete work-up. When autoimmune disorders develop in association with a cancerous process, they are termed *paraneoplasic syndromes.* The rheumatologist does not want to treat the autoimmune disorder with immunosuppressive medications or delay a correct diagnosis if the cause is actually a cancer. This is another factor that adds to the difficulty and time in working with autoimmune disorders.

There are other diagnoses that should be ruled out. Because she has muscle pain, she could have *myositis* (muscle inflammation) or *myopathy* (muscle pathology). She has extreme symptoms of fatigue, which could indicate chronic fatigue syndrome, a chronic viral process. Or the fatigue can be present as part of an autoimmune/inflammatory disorder. She is under stress.

After careful consultation involving well-planned time, a thorough past history, a physical examination, and diagnostic tests, Alice's doctor diagnoses her with Sjögren's syndrome. While hearing that she has a chronic autoimmune disease is not good news for Alice, after a long process of visits to her doctor and specialists, testing to rule out other illnesses, and diagnostics to look for autoimmunity, her diagnosis is a relief. Finally, she knows the reason behind her pain, fatigue, and dryness and can start fighting back against the symptoms that have disturbed her for so long. Like any patient learning she has SjS, Alice will discover that her diagnosis is just the beginning of her understanding of the disease. By working with her doctors and through her own study, she can learn to cope with her symptoms and bring her body and emotions back to balance.

Checklist

What to look for in a physician:
- ☐ will allow one hour for first meeting
- ☐ will follow patient's history carefully
- ☐ will perform a targeted physical examination
- ☐ will order the appropriate blood tests
- ☐ will set an appointment date for discussion of results

Checklist

How to be a good patient:
- ☐ will prepare a written chronological history
- ☐ will collect genetic family history
- ☐ will prepare a list of all medications
- ☐ will have a list of questions with the most significant at the top

3

You, Your Doctor, and Sjögren's Syndrome

AT THIRTY-NINE, FRANCES WAS A BIT OF A JUG-gler. Being a parent to her four children while traveling and managing a large advertising agency, she was vitalized and active but had little time for solitude or rest. What's more, she was going through a divorce. With all of this, it wasn't surprising that she caught every bug around. One morning, after a particularly bad bout of flu, she woke to find that she couldn't stand on the ball of her right foot; it seemed to be without strength.

What followed was a twenty-year odyssey searching for a diagnosis. She couldn't wear fashionable shoes nor could she walk without that quirky foot drag, and worse still was the icy-cold feeling in her right leg and foot. She sought help from every medical specialty that related to legs and feet.

The neurologists agreed that her sensory nerve conduction had been harmed and that there was little question about damage to the nerves of this foot. They could offer no reason for the onset or any suggestion for relief. It was agreed that she indeed had suffered a "foot drop." The orthopedic surgeon injected her back with papain (an enzyme that breaks down scar tissue that could have been contributing to her pain), a particularly painful procedure that was done with a local anesthetic, which produced no change. The rehabilitation specialist diagnosed post-polio syndrome and had her fitted with a cumbersome leg brace.

Over the years, the cold and burning sensation of her leg and foot gradually grew worse. Her symptoms increased. She suffered unbearable fatigue. Her eyes grew dry. The ophthalmologist suggested blepharitis (inflammation of the eyelids) and prescribed eye soaks and cortisone ointment to heal the crusts that formed on her eyes each morning. And still no glimmer of a diagnosis for this increasingly troublesome constellation of symptoms.

Her life became chaotic. Her work suffered and so, too, her feeling of self-worth. The symptoms were many and inconsistent with anything her doctor knew. In that hazy zone where physical and mental health interface, her family doctor capitulated and referred her for psychological evaluation. There seemed little question in his mind and in that of the other doctors that this patient was malingering and that, if she would get meaningfully busy and involved in life, the symptoms would disappear. She sought solace in psychotherapy. While it provided support, it left the underlying problem unresolved.

What was causing it? And what could she do about it? As her frustration mounted, she became increasingly depressed. Until one day a caring neurologist took the time to confer with colleagues, and together, suspecting vasculitis/Sjögren's syndrome (SjS), they referred her to a rheumatologist.

While it may appear that Frances was shuttled around by apathetic, uncaring doctors or that somehow she was responsible, the blame lay with the unfamiliar nature of her disease. Autoimmune diseases, and SjS in particular, pose a diagnostic puzzle for both doctor and patient. The symptoms can take years to develop fully. The disorder is systemic and can cause symptoms anywhere in the patient's body. Most doctors do not have adequate training in the intricacies of diagnosis for a patient with autoimmune disease. Furthermore, managed care does not allow the time for a doctor to really ponder the case thoughtfully before moving on to the next patient.

Why Did It Take So Long to Diagnose?

Like Alice's story in the previous chapter, Frances's story will sound familiar to any rheumatologist and to many who have struggled with undiagnosed SjS. Patients often seek answers for years before receiving a diagnosis. The Sjögren's Syndrome Foundation, in a survey of members (1999), reported that 75 percent of those who responded had a five-year lapse between first symptom and diagnosis. Some took twelve or more years. Considering that studies have shown that early intervention helps in preventing complications, this lapse is clearly harmful.

It's the Nature of the Syndrome

Because SjS is a disorder that takes years to develop, each symptom is often looked upon as unique or isolated and is treated without regard to any others. Checking sinus infections or repeated eye infections restricts the search and obscures the real disorder. It's not unusual for a person to seek help from a physician who specializes in the "broken part." If the symptom is remedied, the search stops. But in the case of an autoimmune disease, the symptoms will not disappear. They persist until the systemic nature of the disorder is properly diagnosed.

In Frances's case, her physicians wanted to help. Each tried specialized tests and treatments. It was the narrowness of their approach that failed her. The neurologist did diagnose the leg weakness and burning pain as small-fiber neuropathy, but he did not speculate on the cause of the neuropathy or on the reason for the cold leg. The icy-cold feeling of the affected leg suggests a vascular involvement, that the oxygen-laden blood was not getting to the nerve tissue. By looking closely at the nerves and their action in her body, the neurologist missed the larger picture.

The orthopedic surgeon, too, jumped to the wrong conclusion. He tried a back injection in case the leg pain came from her spine. It didn't, and Frances suffered a lengthy recovery from the procedure itself.

The rehabilitation doctor tried a leg brace, suspecting a variant of post-polio syndrome. But since neither the back nor polio was the cause, the treatments failed, and Frances dragged the extra weight of the metal brace for months.

The ophthalmologist diagnosed blepharitis and prescribed cortisone ointment. Dry eyes, although common in other conditions such as menopause and allergies, are a direct clue to primary or secondary SjS. The decrease in the volume and quality of normal tears, which contain protective substances against infection, may lead to eye infections like blepharitis. However, the immunosuppressive cortisone ointment, while benefiting in the short term, could add a risk of further infection later on.

And finally, she was referred for psychological assessment and help. Patients like Frances who spend fruitless hours seeking answers often end up in the psychologist's office, having fallen into a clinical depression. Doctors prescribe antidepressants, SSRIs (selective serotonin reuptake inhibitors) such as Prozac, Paxil, and others that, while known to relieve depression, also have physical side effects. For SjS patients, they can aggravate the "dryness" symptoms and make the treatment worse than the disease.

Apart from the diminution of hope that happens after each failed attempt to treat symptom flares, certain treatments can cause harm. Painkillers cause stomach and intestinal bleeding; cortisone ointment leaves the body susceptible to infection; and a heavy leg brace on a weakened, painful leg not receiving enough blood flow can restrict blood flow even further.

With time, Frances developed other symptoms. When she experienced "unbearable" fatigue, doctors attributed it to depression or a busy lifestyle. But the profoundly debilitating fatigue that accompanies autoimmune conditions is often unlike any fatigue the patient has ever experienced.

So, time passed for Frances. And with time, the constellation of symptoms eventually began to form a complete picture. She had burning legs and feet, fatigue, dryness, and pain. With hindsight, we can wonder why it wasn't recognized sooner. Perhaps it is due to rushed doctors, or a patient who didn't realize the need to become a strong advocate for her own care.

New Understanding Brings New Hope

Today's patient can learn about her disorder, how to advocate for herself, and the necessity of forming a partnership with her doctor. Regardless of where on the continuum of care you are—undiagnosed, just diagnosed, or a long-term diagnosed patient—there is an obligation for patients as well as doctors. The patient must always be organized and forthcoming. The patient is not only her symptoms; she is also the composite of her life's story, her work and home, her stress and contentment, all of which contribute to her health. And since managed care allows barely enough consulting time, it becomes even more important for the patient to be clear in her presentation. Instead of stressing only those symptoms that are most troubling at the time, it is important to reveal them all, no matter how trivial they may seem. If a doctor does not have the time or interest in these things, it would be wise to get a second opinion or change doctors.

In Frances's case, stress was a major player in the development of her disease. With all those balls in the air as a manager and creative executive, a mother and homemaker, it is not surprising that one of them dropped. It's too bad it was her health. It's well known that stress contributes to autoimmune disease. Autoimmune disease occurs when there is an imbalance in one's normal immune system. The immune system is constantly alert for stress and infectious agents. Constant vigilance will trigger the immune system too often. Much in the way that viral infections occur more frequently during periods of stress, autoimmunity may be the same, just lasting longer. Furthermore, various infectious agents, even after they are gone, are known to trigger autoimmunity. So even though we cannot prove that stress and frequent infections started her down the road to autoimmunity, it would be fair to speculate that this is so. Frances's list of complaints would include her symptoms of burning legs and feet, fatigue, dryness, and pain. She would include her past infections and how they were treated. She would explain her lifestyle. With these, and a listening physician, she should get a referral to a rheumatologist.

Managing Medical Care

Once Frances received her diagnosis, it became essential for her, as it would be for you, to take stock and become an active partner in her ongoing care. Ask yourself several questions. Which doctor will handle the general care? Which specialist will work best? How comfortable is the relationship between you and your doctor? What do you expect from the partnership? How will you communicate?

Some patients have found that a sympathetic doctor who is willing to learn about the disorder works best for them. Others prefer a physician who, even if not warm and supportive, is knowledgeable and a specialist in autoimmunity. And there are those lucky patients who find both qualities—empathy and skill—in one practitioner.

So, assess your feelings about your caretakers. Which kind of physician are you currently working with? What do you want? Do you want a physician with whom you can talk openly or one who understands the disease but is a little brusque? Perhaps your doctor has a friendly office staff who make your visits more comfortable, and this is important to you. Be aware of your feelings, discuss them with your partner or close friend, and make a careful decision.

If one or another of your physicians is not the best you can find, choose another. If you have a comfortable relationship with a doctor who may not be familiar enough with your disease, you can help her or him learn. Many physicians will appreciate the information you can give them from journal articles, this book, or items from the Internet that they can read and discuss with you. But if your doctor doesn't satisfy your needs it is best to find someone who does. One of the hardest parts of this disorder is believing in the evaluation of your own symptoms and finding a physician who is willing to work with you to define and refine your judgments. Believe in yourself. If you hurt, trust the feeling; it's real. If your doctor won't listen, change doctors. This is a long-term illness; you will want to nurture the relationship with your caretakers for a long-term partnership.

WHAT PHYSICIANS DO YOU NEED?

Each physician you work with must be knowledgeable about SjS or be willing to learn more about it in order to respond to your needs. Every symptom could be related to your disorder regardless of where it occurs in your body. It is not good enough to be referred to a specialist every time something goes wrong. Fragmented care results in frustration for the patient and insufficient information for the physician. You will still need to see certain specialists like your ophthalmologist to obtain the most up-to-date medical treatment and information for your eyes. Some patients will need to take charge as the manager of their own specialists' visits and communicate new information to their general physician, while others will rely completely on their general physician to coordinate their care.

General health: A primary-care or family doctor who understands the impact of SjS on the patient's general health, and who can treat common symptoms and infections, perform tests, and manage the patient's overall care

Autoimmune care: Rheumatologist

Gynecological care: Gynecologist

Eye care: Ophthalmologist

Oral care: Dentist and dental hygienist

Other specialties as symptoms arise

What to Expect from a Doctor

A survey of members of the SjS Foundation in 2001 found most of them wanting a doctor who is patient and thoughtful; who listens and explains things clearly; who treats each patient with respect; who responds by telephone, fax, or e-mail when needed; who, from the beginning, will encourage the patient to contact her or him; and who will explain whether or not there will be extra charges for these communications.

What Your Doctor Expects from You

Since this is a partnership, your physician also has the right to have expectations. You should arrive at your appointments with a written list of symptoms and developments that have occurred since the last visit as well as any medications that have been added by other physicians. Rather than arriving with a vague list of troubles and expecting your doctor to put them together, you should be able to tell your doctor what specifically initiated your visit. Writing things down will help ensure that you don't forget anything once you get to the doctor's office, and it will encourage you to be confident and forthcoming in what can be a stressful situation. Be honest and thoughtful in your disclosures; a partial story is never helpful.

Prioritize your complaints, making sure to list the most troubling one first. Often patients leave the most disturbing complaint until the consultation is almost finished, allowing very little time to sort through the implications and treatment options. Think carefully about what you need to learn from your visit and put that question first. If it's your dry eyes or mouth, muscle pain, fatigue, or wakefulness at night, mention this first.

Be prepared at your visits and take results of any lab tests, X-rays, or reports along with a history of your health. If you need help organizing this information, use our "Patient's Preparation Sheet" on pages 40–41. Also remember to take an extra pad of paper to record any information your doctor gives you. Better still, take a friend to listen and note the information about treatment and prescriptions. Another pair of ears will be a big help.

You should also try to be understanding of your doctor. The very thing that you appreciate—her willingness to spend time with patients who need her—can make her late for your appointment. The pressures on today's doctors are intense; an understanding patient can do a lot to help the partnership.

PATIENT'S PREPARATION SHEET

Filling out a comprehensive information sheet prior to your visits to the doctor can help make the most of the clinician's time with you. The questionnaire below will help you prepare for your appointments. You can copy it and fill it in before your doctor visits. File this after each visit, and you will have a useful history of your disease, its progress, and the various treatments that have been used.

Making qualitative assessments about ourselves and our symptoms is often difficult. It is important to be as specific as possible when consulting with your doctor. To help describe your pain, try these words:

Burning	Pounding	Cramplike
On the surface	Tight	Electric
Sharp	Crushing	Stabbing
Throbbing	Pressing	Pinching
Pulsing	Dull	Pins and needles
Prickling	Shooting	Deep
Stretching	Tender	Gnawing
	Sore	

It is also helpful to your doctor if you can quantitatively rate your pain so that both of you can judge whether your pain is improving or worsening. Use the face scale below to choose a face that best describes the level of pain you are having. Use the number beneath it to give it a rating that you and your doctor can understand.

Faces Pain Scale

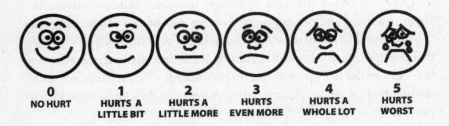

0	1	2	3	4	5
NO HURT	HURTS A LITTLE BIT	HURTS A LITTLE MORE	HURTS EVEN MORE	HURTS A WHOLE LOT	HURTS WORST

PERSONAL HEALTH HISTORY

Your doctor will also need to know your personal health history. Often, you must fill out history forms when you see a new doctor. It will be helpful to you and your doctor if you have a written history prepared prior to your visit, so that you don't forget any important information. Your health history form should include:

- A list of hospitalizations, the dates, and the conditions that took you there
- A list of surgeries, the dates, and the outcomes
- A list of illnesses, the dates, and the outcomes
- A list of allergies
- A list of immunizations (shots): polio, pneumonia, influenza, diphtheria/tetanus, measles, mumps, chicken pox, hepatitis A or B
- A list of medicines/supplements and their amounts
- Family members, ages, and their state of health
- A list of pregnancies, ob/gyn, and hormonal problems
- A list of other health-care providers

Keep a copy of this history, attach it to your Patient's Preparation Sheet, and take it with you for every doctor visit. It can save time and help avoid confusion.

KEEPING IN TOUCH WITH YOUR DOCTOR

Consumer Reports (January 2002) suggests the time has come for e-mail communication between physicians and their patients. At first glance, this sounds practical; however, there are some concerns. Consideration must be made for the privacy of your personal records, the potential for mistakes, and liability for the physician. There is also the possibility of abuse by patients, but, in our opinion, if used carefully and with prudence, e-mail could help alleviate many of the pressures patients and doctors are experiencing in this managed-care environment. E-mail could be used to:

- confirm patient and doctor appointments
- improve access to care
- help patients manage their own care

Patient's Preparation Sheet*

Name: _____ Date: _____

I. The result of our last consultation was: _____
_____

II. The symptoms troubling me today: When it began:

1. _____   _____

2. _____   _____

3. _____   _____

4. _____   _____

5. _____   _____

6. _____   _____

III. Description of my pain: _____
_____

Relief from pain comes when I: _____

IV. The prescription medications I take: Amount:

1. _____   _____

2. _____   _____

3. _____   _____

4. _____   _____

The over-the-counter medications I take: Amount:

1. _____   _____

2. _____   _____

3. _____   _____

4. _____   _____

The alternative medications/nutritional supplements I take: Amount:

1. _____   _____

2. _____   _____

3. _____   _____

4. _____   _____

V. My questions for the doctor:

Q: What do I need to be aware of as I watch the progress of my symptoms?

A: _____

_____

Q: What do I need to know about my medications?

A: _____

_____

Q: What and when is the best way to contact you? Telephone? E-mail? Fax?

A: _____

_____

Q: When should I make a follow-up appointment?

A: _____

_____

Q: _____

A: _____

_____

Q: _____

A: _____

_____

*Attached is my "Health History."

E-mail could be used by doctors to communicate uncomplicated and standard test results and by patients to request medications. It can facilitate doctor-to-patient communication of education materials, appointment reminders, and general office administration announcements. In fact, one physician reported that he keeps a list of e-mail addresses of consenting patients and after September 11, 2001, was able to communicate with them while his office, which was close to the World Trade Center, was closed for seven days.

Nonetheless, there are privacy problems to be considered. Messages are permanent and easily accessible, and thus vulnerable to being altered, forwarded, or otherwise distributed throughout the Internet. The physician could misspell the name of a medication or misplace a digit in the dosage, and a pharmacist may be less likely to question a typed note than a handwritten one. Furthermore, the urgency of patient-to-doctor communication or vice versa may be lost if either reads her or his e-mail only once a day. E-mail makes the recipient responsible for monitoring the computer twenty-four hours a day or risk possible endangerment.

With the caveat that e-mail should never be used for an emergency situation and with awareness of privacy considerations, it is possible to use e-mail to improve patient relations and to decrease the pressure on the doctor's office staff for run-of-the-mill management. Ask your doctor if she would enter into an agreement with you so that, for a fee, you could communicate with her by e-mail. Set the parameters for these communications at the same time that you set the fee. Ask if her e-mail system has privacy features so you can protect yourself. Check whether anyone else in the office has access to the messages and write with this in mind. And consider sending these messages only from your home address and never from your work.

E-mail is not for diagnosis or opinions. It is perfect for confirming appointments, requesting information on the side effects of medications, checking in after the doctor has given a medication, asking a simple question, or keeping her up-to-date on a past visit.

If your physician is overwhelmed at the thought of e-mails flowing in from all her patients and would prefer that you telephone, that's fine. You might also ask if she would prefer a fax of simple questions to a telephone call. Whatever you choose, make sure that you and your doctor have an understanding you're both comfortable with.

Take Charge!

These few ideas are included to remind us all that it is the patient's responsibility to take control of her care and the physician's responsibility to listen, diagnose, and treat the illness. The time is gone when we could deliver ourselves to the caring family doctor and have her solve our problems. Medicine now is more complex. But with this change has come an exponential growth in our knowledge of medicine and the ways in which it can improve our quality of life. Each of us can be an advocate for our own health. Be prepared and keep track of changes, medications, and symptoms so that the medical visit will yield positive and helpful results.

CHAPTER 4

Dry Eyes

ON A BRIGHT SUNNY DAY, WHEN A NEIGHBOR ASKS you to keep an eye on the kids while she runs to the corner store, you drop everything and gladly step outside to help. You do that, that is, if your eyes are not inflamed and have normal tearing capacity. If you suffer from the dry eyes of Sjögren's syndrome (SjS), you will need to think twice, and then you will likely decline. Your eyes hurt in the sun. At the best of times they burn, sting, and sometimes exude a discharge, but in the bright light of the sun, the pain is unbearable. For some reason, bright light makes you squint and want to close your eyes.

Dry eyes call attention to themselves. They hurt, so you blink, but the blinking brings little relief. The feeling gets worse as the day goes on. Working at a computer becomes increasingly difficult. The normal, everyday environment of most people—air-conditioning in a home, a windy day, a fan in your office, dry air on an airplane—are problems for you. You use eye drops—the ones to get the "redness" out—and they make your eyes worse. You try others, specifically designed for dry eyes, and they help relieve the burning for a while.

Dry eyes are not a minor inconvenience; they are painful and can interfere with your quality of life, even with your livelihood. What's more, they are costly. Researchers associated with Harvard Medical School and Tufts University of Dental Medicine estimate that the cost of dry-eye treatments for an individual with SjS is in excess of $300 "out of pocket" each year.

Those not diagnosed with SjS but who experience this painful symptom should search for an ophthalmologist who specializes in dry eyes. She can test your eyes and ask questions about medications, history, reaction to your surroundings, and allergies. Since dryness in the eyes increases in everyone as we age, she will look to see if this is age-related dryness. Some medications, such as diuretics, some antihistamines, decongestants, certain hormones, tricyclic antidepressants, and certain acne medications, can cause dryness. Because of irritants and diminished moisture in the air, eyes can become dry when the air is smog filled. Eyes can become dryer at menopause. Staring at a computer screen for long periods seriously lowers the rate at which you blink, which in turn causes dry eyes. Any of these should cause you to seek a doctor's advice. She will question you and, when all of the other factors are ruled out, she will move on to assess the possibility of autoimmunity and SjS.

What Is Happening to Make My Eyes Dry?

It may surprise you to learn that everyone at one time or another suffers from dry eyes. Fifty percent of those over sixty-five experience dry eyes, a condition that worsens with time. The degree of suffering varies from person to person as do the suggested reasons for it. It is not an affliction with one cause.

Keratoconjunctivitis sicca (KCS) or dry eye can be subdivided into two groups. While both groups experience dry eyes in varying degrees, the root cause of the dryness is different. Basically, the distinction is made based on the appearance of inflammation, or the lack thereof. Eyes without obvious signs of inflammation may, for certain reasons not related to

It makes me mad when my friends don't realize how painful dry eyes are. Sometimes when I tell them about the dryness, they nod and smile and think they are helping by saying "We understand. We get dry eyes too." Then, they move on to the next bit of gossip. Aghhh! They don't really understand! We are not talking about a bit of dry eyes off and on. SjS folks have it constantly. I have to wet my eyes all during the day and even at night, so I never get a good night's sleep.

—Debra

SjS, not react as they should. Common irritants that cause dry, burning, and itchy eyes are:

- smoky environments that make it difficult for your tears to clear noxious substances
- allergies
- chemicals in an enclosed space
- dry, recycled air, such as that in airplanes or air-conditioned offices
- inability of your eyelids to close completely due to poor cosmetic surgery or Graves' thyroid disease
- computer work that keeps your eyes open without blinking for an extended period

Such environmental, mechanical, and anatomical conditions can cause KCS. By adding moisture back to the eye in the form of artificial tears, you can feel relief. People with irritated eyes probably account for approximately 15 percent of those over sixty-five in the United States who have dryness symptoms.

Unlike irritated eyes, the eyes of SjS patients are dry as a result of inflammation caused by a systemic condition. Inflammation in the eye causes many changes. There can be:

- a decrease in the mucin-secreting cells
- increased permeability of the cornea
- decrease in the production of tears
- the release of *cytokines,* small protein molecules that serve as messengers between cells, regulating cell activity through interaction with special cell-surface receptors

Any of the foregoing can lead to symptoms of KCS. Inflammation accounts for the dry-eye complaints of 2 to 16 percent of patients over sixty-five. They can be helped somewhat by adding artificial tears to wash out the debris. The effect of adding tears is not so much to add liquid to the eye but rather to wash away the dead cells and cytokines. That explains why, after artificial tears are added, their beneficial effect gradually diminishes and you need to add more, sometimes as soon as one hour later. These added tears have washed away the waste, but more has accumulated.

Tears

Simple as they appear, tears are a complex film with three layers that originates in a separate gland. The watery liquid that we think of as tears is produced in the lacrimal glands, located under the upper eyelid. This liquid is sandwiched between two gooey layers: the mucous layer on the inside and the oily layer on the outside. The mucous layer is secreted from the goblet cells on the eye surface; it helps the tear film adhere to the eye. The oily viscous layer is secreted by the meibomian glands along the bottom of the eye opening; it prevents the tear from evaporating into the air.

This three-layered tear film is essential for vision; it lubricates and protects the surface, has antimicrobial properties, flushes away debris and microorganisms, provides surface cells with oxygen and metabolites, and delivers immune cells to sites of injury or infection.

Everyone with dry eyes will suffer for one of three reasons:

- a problem with the secretion of tears,
- a problem with the components of the tears themselves, or
- tears that evaporate from the eye surface too quickly.

The symptoms of burning or pain are the result of increased friction as the eyelid passes over the eye surface without sufficient lubrication, much like a windshield wiper without fluid. In normal eyes, the lid movements are helped by the tear film. In dry eyes, abnormalities in any or all of the three causes—the secretions, components, or hyperevaporation—will cause dry-eye symptoms.

Additionally, inflammatory substances accumulate in the eye and directly irritate the tissues. As well as making it physically difficult for your eyelid to oscillate, surface abrasions can develop if the dryness is not attended to early enough. Further damage can result when a resulting corneal abrasion or ulcer gets infected.

In the past, it was believed that the lacrimal gland, the gland that dispenses the aqueous layer of the tear film, became inflamed and secreted fewer tears onto the eye. With new research findings, we are learning that eye dryness can happen in stages and that each stage is associated with a different effect that requires different treatment. If your eyes are in the early stage of dryness, a simple tear substitute might help. Once your eyes

---

The Four Stages of Eye Dryness

1. Loss of water from the tear film, resulting in a concentration of other tear components.
2. Decrease in the cells that secrete mucin.
3. Increase in cellular debris on the surface of the eye.
4. Destabilization of the cornea-tear interface, resulting in decreased corneal cell surface.

---

are further compromised (which is inevitable for SjS patients), a complex tear-replacement regimen or procedure may be called for.

Recently, the above summary has been expanded to include an understanding that the most troubling form of KCS is due to inflammatory substances in the tear film and on the surface of the eye itself. These inflammatory substances are the same small protein molecules known to be involved in the inflammatory response in other diseased tissues, such as the *synovial* (joint) fluid of rheumatoid arthritis patients. Cytokines are currently being investigated as major players in inflammatory disorders. This knowledge has a major implication in treatment choices, as you will see.

BLEPHARITIS

Blepharitis, a common complication of SjS, is inflammation of the eyelids. Its symptoms are worse in the morning when you awaken. At times, your eyes are sealed shut, have crusty yellow bits adhering to them, and often have small bumps like styes on the lid margin. This disorder is thought to result from an oozing and congealing of the secretions of the *meibomian glands* along the rims of the eyelids. It is common in those with dry eyes and can be worsened by the thick eye drops or heavy face cream some of us use before sleeping. Steady treatment with hot compresses and massage each morning is the first approach to helping clear up the condition (see below). If heat and washing don't help enough, see your ophthalmologist for more intensive therapy with steroids and antibiotics. Continue the scrubs and hot compresses even after the symptoms have gone. It will ensure the condition does not return. Remember that wiping or rubbing your eye could cause pathogens to enter and create infection. Keeping your hands away is the first step to eye health. If you need to rub, do so gently with a clean tissue, never a used one.

Medications That Can Cause Dry Eyes	
Category	**Drug Name**
Diuretics	hydrochlorothiazide
Antihistamines	Benadryl
	Chlor-Tripilon
	Claritin
	Zyrtec
	Allegra
	pseudoephedrine
	phenylpropanolamine
Antidepressants	Prozac
	Elavil
Acne Medications	Accutane
Anti-Anxiety Medications	Librium
	Valium
Hormones /Oral Contraceptives	estrogens
	progestins/combinations
Antispasmodic	Bentyl

Eye Tests

The physician will begin by looking at your eyes to assess the state of the tear film. A careful examination through a slit-lamp biomicroscope will give a three-dimensional view of the eye's surface and show tear quality, quantity, and surface damage. The doctor will look for debris or mucin and signs of inflammation on the eye as well as under the lower lid.

Schirmer's Test

The doctor will also perform a simple Schirmer's test. The Schirmer's test will ascertain if the lacrimal gland is producing tears and of what volume (the quantity during a specific time) they are. During this test, filter-paper strips about ½" x 1½" are placed gently under the lower eyelids lengthwise. The volume of tear flow from the lacrimal gland is measured by how many milliliters of the paper strip are moistened in five minutes. Most people produce 8 milliliters of tear flow in five minutes. Less than 5 milliliters is associated with a clinically significant decrease in tearing. Although topical anesthetics are not recommended for a Schirmer's test, if you are given one before the test, be aware that your result will be lower than that from a test done without it.

In another Schirmer's test, the doctor will insert a cotton swab into the nose to stimulate the lacrimal gland and repeat the test. It is very important at this stage to ascertain whether or not the lacrimal glands are producing any tears. If the doctor sees signs that your eyes have some tearing potential, she will make a note of that for treatment possibilities. The Schirmer's test alone is not enough to diagnose KCS.

Rose Bengal or Fluorescein Test

Another test for tear quality is to check the fluorescence of rose bengal or fluorescein when they are applied to the eye. Rose bengal and fluorescein are vegetable dyes that are instilled in the eye to outline any dry spots on the eye surface. Both dyes are used to measure tear volume and outline the spots that have eroded because of dryness. Fluorescein spots correlate directly with the amount of discomfort patients experience. Fluorescein is used to determine "tear breakup time" or how well your tears maintain their integrity. With your eyes open, the doctor will add the dye and take note of the time it takes for the tears to evaporate and to see dry spots on the cornea. Because it stings and can be irritating to dry eyes, rose bengal is now often replaced with fluorescein.

Treatment

Dry eyes need to be watched and monitored in order to avoid serious complications. They can be treated, but before treatment they must be diagnosed to differentiate between the possible causes. While there are diagnostic tests, a doctor's experience is crucial to making accurate medical judgments. You will need to find a qualified ophthalmologist who has had experience with the vagaries of dry eyes. To do this, you can contact the American Medical Association or the equivalent medical association in your country and inquire with your own HMO or medical group. Since there is no specialty designated for "dry eye," look for a board-certified cornea specialist.

Your symptoms will tell the doctor much about the condition of your eyes. If your complaint includes a chronic state of sandy or gritty discomfort and you report that it worsens as the day goes by, she will begin to think about KCS. If your eyes are more troublesome in the morning and clear up as the day goes on, she will look to see if your eyelids are inflamed and if so, begin to investigate the possibility of blepharitis.

Once you are diagnosed with dry eyes, you will find it is important to maintain a regular schedule of visits with your ophthalmologist. Serious eye conditions require careful medical attention. Severe dry eye is associated with the adherence of mucus and debris on the eye surface, known as *filamentary keratosis*. It can be avoided but only with the regular attention of an ophthamologist. You and your doctor should decide how often you will need to be seen, and you should keep to the timetable; your eyes change often, so they need tender loving care and watchfulness.

Currently, there is no cure for dry eyes. Until we uncover the mechanism that triggers the infiltration of lymphocytes into the moisture-producing glands and are able to interfere with the process, a cure remains unlikely. But, tools to manage the symptoms are improving. There are prescription medications, over-the-counter medications and treatment aids, and home remedies. Relief can come from a varying array of treatments, including humidifiers, special moisture-retaining glasses, improved tear substitutes, lubricating ointments, lubricating inserts, medications, and surgical interventions.

Artificial Tears

Artificial tears are the foundation of dry eye treatment, but they do not heal dry eyes; they provide comfort when used throughout the day. There are more than thirty different artificial tear products on the market, some with preservatives in multiuse bottles, some without preservatives in single-

Why Can't I Wear Contacts?

Contact lenses, particularly soft contact lenses, absorb moisture from the eye and are very uncomfortable for anyone with dry eyes. They can contribute to corneal abrasions because if there is not an adequate supply of tears to wash away the debris, the debris gets trapped under the lens. Still, if you need to wear contact lenses and your condition allows you to do so without pain, it is wise to instill preservative-free artificial tears often to wash your eye.

People don't like to be noticed doing something unusual like constantly putting drops in their eyes. But the fact is, we need the tears. Henrietta in Norfolk, Virginia, told us she got past her embarrassment when she saw a young woman at the races using artificial tears. When she asked, the woman explained that her contacts were bothering her. She thought nothing of adding tears! Henrietta realized that her shame came from some deeply held belief that her condition somehow made her inferior. She sought therapy because the worry and concern became too heavy for her to bear. In the therapist's office, she was able to feel compassion for herself and gradually gained the strength to realize that she had much in her life besides her disorder. Slowly, her image of herself turned around, and she became comfortable with the idea that adding drops to her eyes in public was what allowed her to do the things she enjoyed. Today she accepts her need to look after herself. She blithely adds drops to her eyes whenever she needs them and finds her friends take little notice.

use droppers. Some are viscous while others are clear. Recently, Allergan announced the arrival of a new prescription artificial tear product, Restasis, which has been approved by the Food and Drug Administration for use to increase tear production. But more on that later. Most over-the-counter tear solutions are formulated similarly. One brand has bicarbonate added, another has simple saline and still others use electrolyte concentrations and buffers that give the "tears" a longer-lasting effect.

The only way to know which artificial tear will suit you is to try them. Your physician may be able to guide you as to which she thinks might work for you.

Artificial tears can be divided into three subcategories:

1. artificial tears with preservatives in multidose bottles
2. artificial tears without preservatives found in single-use containers
3. lubricating ointmentlike artificial tears that are thicker and more viscous found in single- and multiuse containers

Artificial Tears with Preservatives

Some preservatives found in artificial tears can cause an allergic reaction that leads to itching or can become toxic to the ocular surface and cause irritation and inflammation. Some artificial tears with preservatives are:

- GenTeal Mild or Moderate (Novartis)
- Refresh Tears (Allergan)
- Tears Plus (Allergan)
- Hypotears (Novartis)
- Tears Naturale II (Alcon)

Preservative-Free Artificial Tears

Patients who require artificial tears more than four times a day will prefer to use preservative-free artificial tear formulations. Preservative-free artificial tears are also based on hydroxypropyl methylcellulose but are packed in single-use vials. They are meant to be used just once, not kept for later use; any residual amount left in them should be thrown away. Preservative-free artificial tears include:

- Refresh Lubricant or Liquijel or PM (Allergan)
- GenTeal Gel (Novartis)
- Hypotears PF (IOLAB)
- Lacri-Lube (Allergan)

Ointments

The various artificial lubricants available for dry-eye treatment also have a range of viscosity. In patients with more severe dry-eye symptoms, an artificial-tear ointment or gel at bedtime helps to provide lubrication throughout the night. These ointments tend to blur vision and therefore have limited usefulness during the day. Sometimes these thicker preparations can clog the meibomian glands, in which case you should remember to use the hot compress and cleaning system we describe on page 59. Common ointment treatments include:

- Celluvisc (Allscripts)
- Refresh PM (Allergan)
- Moisture Eyes PM (Bausch & Lomb) (formerly Duolube)

New Tear Formulations

Early in 2003, the Food and Drug Administration approved a new prescription dry-eye therapy, sold as Restasis. It is formulated to control inflammation and restore tear-producing cells to their more natural state. In clinical trials using the Schirmer's wetting test (the test that measures the dryness of your eyes), Restasis, an Allergan product, was proven to significantly increase tears over a six-month period. Your doctor will be able to discuss it in detail with you.

Two new artificial-tear products in the United States and one in Canada have duplicated more precisely the nature of our natural tears. All three are worth trying if the others have not been effective. They maintain an electrolyte balance that mimics human tear film and are less concentrated. They allow water to move back into the eye to relieve symptoms and restore balance. The brands available in the United States are Bion Tears (Alcon) and TheraTears (Advanced Vision Research), which use bicarbonate, a component of natural tears. Eyestil (Ophthapharma/Canada), available in Canada, uses sodium hyaluronate, a formulation with anti-inflammatory action.

For those with moderate to severe dry eyes, gels, which are new preparations that are more viscous than tears but lighter than ointments, may provide relief. Such products include Tears Again Gel, Refresh Liquigel, and Refresh Endura, a brand-new tear formulation that is an emulsion more viscous than tears but even less so than a gel. The active ingredient is suspended in an emulsion. Check with your ophthalmologist about any of these new products and their use in your condition.

Lacrisert (Merck) is a time-released insert for your eye that slips moisture over the surface. It is composed of sterilized hydroxypropyl methylcellulose. These tiny plastic pellets of concentrated artificial tears are tucked under your lower eyelid each day to slowly dissolve and dispense tears over a longer period of time. They can be very useful in treating patients with moderate to severe dry-eye syndrome. However, they tend to blur vision for several hours after insertion. They are difficult for some patients to handle and are significantly more expensive than artificial tears. If your ophthalmologist feels they would be a benefit in your case, he will prescribe them. These inserts were unavailable during the days of Desert Storm because all available stock was sent to the armed forces to avert dry eyes caused by blowing sand. They are now in full supply and available by prescription. Unfortunately, the manufacturer (Merck) has discontinued its practice of allowing patients to try a sample product before purchase, so do discuss their application for your condition with your physician.

Worth Trying . . . If All Else Fails

Designers of artificial tears are constantly seeking to improve their products. Cyclosporin A, for example, has proven successful when instilled into the dry eyes of dogs and has been approved for veterinary medicine. It is used as a steroid-sparing eye drop and can be prepared for you with prescription by a compounding pharmacist.

Another additive that is in use in Canada and Europe is sodium hyaluronate. In clinical trials it has been shown to improve the symptoms and signs of dry-eye syndrome and to improve ocular surface damage. Although expensive, it can be prepared in the United States by a compounding pharmacist.

USING ARTIFICIAL TEARS

When using any artificial tear, be sure to wash your hands first. Keep the drops as germ-free as possible by never allowing the bottle tip to touch your eye. Also keep the bottle as tightly sealed as possible when not using it.

To use, soak your eyes with the fluid, gently close your eyes, and hold them closed for about one minute. Many of the drops are meant to fully saturate the eye surface. After about one minute, gently remove any tears that are left in your lashes or on your cheek. You will feel much better once your eyes have had a chance to soak in the water coating. You will need to experiment to find a routine that works for you.

PUNCTAL OCCLUSION: CONTROL THE TEARS YOU HAVE

If changing the environment and adding tears does not help, you might consider having the drains in your eyes closed. Each eye has two openings or drainage canals, called *puncta* (tear ducts), located in the corner on the top and bottom, near the bridge of the nose. They serve as drains through which tears are washed away into and down the nasal passage. This treatment may be contraindicated if you already produce a fair amount of tears. Once the puncta are closed, tears could overflow and run down your cheeks. On the other hand, if you produce *some* tears but not enough, closing the drains to retain wetness is a logical strategy. The procedure is done in an ophthalmologist's office. Often, patients will need only the lower puncta closed.

Puncta can be stopped up either temporarily or permanently. For tem-

My eyes burn and hurt quite a bit throughout the day. During the day I use single-use drops once every hour, a gel every two hours, and an eye ointment overnight. Until I established this routine, I used ordinary bottled artificial tears, and then I realized that the preservative in them was giving me more pain. Now I have switched to single-use tears with bicarbonate in them and continue with the gel and ointment. They seem to help, along with the humidifier and eye soaks. When we go biking, I wear wraparound eye shields.

—Rosalind

porary closure, collagen or silicone plugs are inserted into the opening. Collagen plugs dissolve and last about two days. Silicon plugs are durable and may be removed if there are excessive tears after the plugs are inserted. In rare cases, the plugs slip out because they are the wrong size. It need not concern you; the physician will check and try a more suitable size. Still, not everyone is comfortable with plugs, perhaps because the inflammatory process has not been tamed. If there is debris in your eye due to inflammation, you may be advised to undergo the steroid treatment we discuss on page 61 before closing the puncta.

By and large, this procedure has given great relief to patients for whom it is appropriate. In a survey of SjS patients chosen at random (Sullivan et al., Schepens Eye Research Institute), 53.3 percent had received punctal occlusion or plugs.

Patients who get satisfying results with plugs often opt for a more permanent treatment. The ophthalmologist will cauterize the puncta or laser them shut. It is a very brief process: You hear a *ping* and sense a pinprick and it is over. Many patients report success with this method, using drops only occasionally. But again, make sure you have your eyes checked regularly, even when they do not feel dry anymore. They can be dry without your being aware that they are. The only way to know is to have them seen by your ophthalmologist.

SYSTEMIC MEDICATIONS

Drugs available in pill form are the "big guns" when it comes to SjS, so most patients prefer to save them for more serious conditions. New treatments for the systemic effects of SjS are being discovered every year, but at present, treatment tends to be palliative—symptoms are treated as they arise.

Some patients report relief with systemic medications. In consultation with your rheumatologist, you may choose to try drugs such as hydroxy-chloroquine (Plaquenil), methotrexate, or azathioprine. They are used to attack inflammation throughout the body, thereby treating the underlying immune process to possibly alleviate the symptoms of dry eyes. Unfortunately, these DMARDs (disease-modifying antirheumatic drugs) are immunosuppressant—they reduce your body's ability to fight disease—and could increase the risk and severity of infections. Using them for dry eyes alone may be something you will want to discuss in detail with your physician.

There are two new medications available for dry mouth that have been shown to help dry eyes as well, although they are not yet approved for this purpose by the Food and Drug Administration. They increase secretions from the exocrine glands, including tears and saliva, by stimulating the muscarinic receptor. The most recent agent, cevimeline (Evoxac), is a 30-mg tablet taken three times a day. The first agent available, pilocarpine hydrochloride (Salagen), is a 5-mg tablet taken four times a day. Although many patients report success with these drugs, each one has some side effects, the most noticeable being increased perspiration and flushing.

A cautionary note: If you have risk factors for heart disease or have asthma, be sure you tell your physician. There is also concern with the development of certain eye conditions such as *iritis,* or narrow-angle glaucoma, so do ask about these in your particular case. And since these medications need to be taken either three or four times each day, it has been reported that compliance tends to be less rigorous than it should be. Compliance is usually better with medicines dosed less frequently. It seems that patients will only use these agents if they have *very* severe symptoms which remind them to take the drugs frequently. Often they are on many other medications and just do not want to take another pill. Don't let these drawbacks stop you from trying them. For those who find them useful, they are "miraculous."

Other drugs are targeted at decreasing inflammation throughout the body or decreasing the autoimmune process itself. Plaquenil (hydroxy-chloroquine) is a mild immunomodulator that can down-regulate pro-inflammatory cytokines like IL-1 and TNF-alpha and therefore often is beneficial. It is a 200-mg tablet that can be taken once a day. The usual dose is 200 to 400 mg per day. In some patients, the higher doses can be "drying" and fail to produce a net beneficial effect. Again, if you remain on hydroxychloroquine, be sure to consult with your ophthalmologist for eye changes at least once a year.

HOME REMEDIES

There are simple things you can do to protect and help your eyes. Think about items that hold moisture in like plastic wrap and wraparound sunglasses. Think about items that bring moisture into your environment like an on-the-desk or room humidifier. For a list of Sjögren's-friendly products, check out the Sjögren's Syndrome Foundation web site (*www.sjogrens.org*) or request the brochure "Product List Directory" from the Foundation offices (301-718-0300). Here are some other suggestions you might like to consider.

Humidify

For those with dry eyes but little tear production, treatment is focused on relieving the symptoms. To prevent evaporation, be sure the environment is not too dry. At the office, a small vaporizer used in a baby's room can sit on your desk or wherever you find you work most often. For your home, there are room and house humidifiers, air washers, and vaporizers. A forced-hot-air furnace is very drying and almost always will require humidification, either for a single room or as an insert into the furnace for the whole house. Even if the price is prohibitive for a whole-house unit, buying a moisture-producing unit is essential for the bedroom. Whichever you

---

Sometimes I Have Too Many Tears!

Barbara in San Carlos, California, couldn't understand it. Her eyes were dry, but sometimes, when she went outside and there was a strong wind, tears ran down her face. It seems contradictory to have dry eyes with too many tears, but it does happen. When your eye is irritated, a stimulus causes your lacrimal glands to produce more water. These tears are responding to a stimulant and are meant to react to that stimulant and then disappear. These *reflex tears* (Cassel et al., *The Eye Book*) that roll down the cheeks when the eye is irritated are not very good quality tears. They are lacking the viscous material (mucins) that holds the tear onto the eye surface and cannot perform the protective duties of regular tears.

choose, make sure to clean it regularly to avoid further pollutants being dispersed into the air and continue to use it throughout the year, not just in winter.

Sunglasses

Wraparound glasses, those with side panels, that are worn either over your eyeglasses or alone, protect your eyes from environmental dryness. Especially when used with artificial tears, these protective eye coverings reduce the effect of wind, air-conditioning, and sudden gusts of air. Some opticians or ophthalmologists will make side shields for your existing glasses to help retain moisture. They decrease the amount of evaporation by keeping circulating air out.

Bright light and sun can be stressful. Upgrade the protective coating on your sunglasses from the standard Polaroid coating to the mirrorlike or reflective coating. It adds cost but helps reduce the glare on the surface of your eye. Wide-brimmed hats can also help in a sun-sensitive environment.

Plastic Wrap

If you find that your eyelids do not close completely when you sleep and that your eyes lose moisture to the atmosphere at night, try sealing them shut with plastic wrap. Use two sheets of plastic wrap, one on top of the other, and secure the wrap to the side of your face and forehead with bandage tape. This will help keep that moisture IN!

Cucumber Slices

Don't overlook the simple things that can help tired, dry eyes. Soothe your eyes by placing a thin cucumber slice over each eye as you rest. To help clear the eye surface, simply close your eyes and roll the eyeball around the whole surface. Compresses, warm and cool, will comfort burning, tired eyes.

Warm Eye Compresses

Set aside a special time each morning when you can place a hot facecloth (as hot as you can stand) over your eyes. To lengthen the time that the cloth stays warm and to minimize dribbles, put a dampened facecloth in an unsealed plastic bag in the microwave oven and microwave for ten to fifteen seconds. Place the heated plastic-enclosed cloth over your eyes and lie down. If the plastic is too hot, remove the cloth and use that alone.

When the compress has cooled, wash your eyes with an eye-cleaning solution. Eye-Scrub (made by Ciba Vision) works well. Some SjS patients use baby shampoo diluted half and half with water, but others find it irritating. Whichever cleaning system works best for you, try to practice this ritual twice every day. To save money and for traveling, dampen several gauze squares with the solution and store them in a small plastic bag; you'll use less.

Modify Your Computer

Computers have changed how we work in many ways. For those with dry eyes it has made them worse, mainly because working at a computer for long periods causes us to forget to blink. In a 1998 research study (Yamada), it was shown that the rate of blinking is significantly decreased while sitting at a computer. Those of us with dry eyes did not need a study to tell us that our eyes are worse at the end of a work day. What we need is the reminder at our elbows to blink as we work. It takes a conscious effort on the patient's part to remember to blink often. And to take breaks. Walk away for a few minutes and change the focus of your eyes. Add artificial tears more often. Be aware that work like this will cause the blink rate to go down. Bring it up—blink!

And consider a special antiglare screen for your computer as well as computer glasses with a tint. Simple measures, it's true, but we have found them to be effective.

Of course, there are those for whom blinking will not work because there aren't enough tears available to coat the eye surface. There are computer programs that will read aloud whatever is entered or scanned in. They are expensive, but often your local disability center can direct you to a source for a more reasonably priced program.

Massage

Another self-treatment that helps inflammation of the meibomian gland is gentle massage twice a day. Use a warm washcloth to gently massage your eyelids for about five seconds, paying special attention to the lower lids. This will increase blood flow to the lids and decrease inflammation.

Eye Goggles

One of the less engaging but useful suggestions is to wear swim goggles when you are planning an outing that could be especially threatening. It

---

Plastic Surgery—Is It Possible?

Eyelids are delicate, as are the pouches beneath the eyes. Nevertheless, there are many who would change them for a better appearance. If handled carefully by a skilled surgeon who is knowledgeable about dry eyes, plastic surgery is possible. Possible, that is, for a person with mild to moderate dryness, and even then the surgery should not be extensive. It is especially important to maintain a full lid to cover the eye. Patients with severe dry eye should probably forgo surgery or consider very conservative changes. The dryness will be more pronounced immediately after surgery but will improve with time.

---

may not be esthetically pleasing, but—hey!—we are talking comfort here. Barz goggles, made in Australia, can be custom ordered in your prescription for outdoor and computer wear.

NEW TREATMENTS ON THE HORIZON

Current research is uncovering new possibilities for the treatment of dry eye. *Androgens* (male hormones) added to an artificial tear have been successful in improving lacrimal gland function and reducing lacrimal gland lymphocytic infiltration in experimental studies.

Eye drops using cyclosporine, sodium hyaluronate, and Vitamin A are being tested, with the hope that with formula refinement, they eventually will be approved for use by the Food and Drug Administration. One, Restasis, the prescription cyclosporine eye drop, was approved by the FDA in early 2003.

A newer treatment for certain kinds of dry eye is based on the presence of inflammatory substances in the tears and on the surface of the eye. As research into dry eye is increasingly pointing to inflammation as the root cause of the condition, anti-inflammatory agents are becoming the remedies of choice. Steroids such as Decadron, which reduce inflammation, can be mixed into an artificial tear medium. When given in pulse doses over a short time and then tapered off, they can lessen the inflammation, allowing tears to flow from the lacrimal gland. Steroid treatment has been shown to have a lasting effect and to remarkably improve the irritation symptoms and ocular signs of KCS. Before beginning this treatment, your physician will need to be certain that you are secreting tears from the lacrimal gland. A quick way to find out whether or not you might be a candidate for this treatment is to ask yourself how you react to freshly chopped onion. If you cry, you will likely benefit. Important note: There is a risk of glaucoma or premature cataracts with extended use of steroids. After a short course of steroids, a patient must be switched to a steroid-sparing agent such as cyclosporin A.

Treat Yourself Well!

Our bodies need replenishing through rest, as do our eyes. Have you thought of giving yourself a regular program of massage? Closing your eyes and surrounding yourself with moist, warm air while a skilled nurturing massage therapist kneads your tired muscles will do wonders for a body that suffers from pain and fatigue and for eyes that are dry. It not only feels good but also contributes to healing. Tension results in increased sympathetic nervous system tone, which results in decreased exocrine secretions. So when you reduce tension, you reduce the call on your sympathetic nervous system.

For daily caring, try audiobooks. Elinor R. of Oakland, California, credits them with keeping her spirits up. We are not promising wonders, but a caring body massage, rest, and a good (audio) book with eyes closed for an hour or so can't help but restore your equilibrium.

CHAPTER 5

Dry Mouth, Nose, and Throat

Dry Mouth

You may never miss the water till the well runs dry, but when it is the saliva in your mouth, you miss it quickly enough. Without saliva, your mouth feels dry and sticky, your tongue can grow thick and painful, and red and white splotches may appear on the mouth's mucosa. Foods that once tasted sumptuous suddenly become bitter or tasteless. You can't swallow dry foods without a sip of water, and there is less saliva in the "pool" below your tongue. You can speak and eat only with sips of water to help moisten your mouth. And your dentist finds a multitude of dental problems.

> About two years before I knew I had Sjögren's syndrome, I went to the dentist. It had been about six months since my last checkup, and yet I had ten cavities! I couldn't understand it because I had never had more than one or two, and those took years to develop. The dentist couldn't tell me why it was happening and simply assumed I had poor dental hygiene. That made me feel awful, but not as bad as when I discovered another seven cavities six months later! Of course, once I had the diagnosis of Sjögren's syndrome, it all became clear.
>
> —Julia

Dry mouth, or *xerostomia,* is not seen in every SjS patient. You can have dry eyes with or without dry mouth and vice versa. But even if you don't suffer from dry mouth now, it does not follow that you never will. It is difficult for anyone who has never experienced the symptoms of dry mouth to fully comprehend the enormous impact of the disorder: the changes in everyday routine, the difficulty in social relationships, the depression it can bring. Nevertheless, there are millions around the world who share this sorrow with you.

Understanding Dry Mouth: Saliva

Saliva is astonishing: It coats our teeth and the foods we eat with a smooth viscous fluid, allowing us to chew and swallow what otherwise would be jagged, irritating hunks of dry material. It cleans our mouth and teeth and protects against bacteria. Mucins (glycoproteins) in saliva help lubricate our mouths when talking, eating, and cheering our favorite little league team and continue to do this whether we are awake or asleep. Saliva also plays a role in the perception of taste. The components of saliva maintain the balance between acidity and alkalinity at a steady neutral state (pH of 7.0). If the pH shifts to become more acidic, as it does with a lack of saliva, plaque forms on our teeth. The bacteria living in plaque will metabolize sugars in our food to create an acidic environment, encouraging swift decay of our teeth as the acid erodes through tooth enamel.

There are proteins (secretory IgA), enzymes (lysozymes and lactoperoxidase), and histatins in our saliva that suppress bacteria, materials that protect the teeth, electrolytes, hormones, and enzymes, all of which aid in keeping our mouths free of infection, dental erosion, and discomfort. Once the moisture is withdrawn, we suffer innumerable problems. Saliva is also important in maintaining the mineralization of the tooth by providing a local source of calcium and phosphate, which precipitate from the healthy foods we eat directly into our saliva.

Saliva is produced by three pairs of salivary glands: the parotid glands, the submandibular glands, and the sublingual glands. The parotid glands, located in front of the ears and down the side of each cheek, release saliva through the cheeks. The submandibular glands are located between the lower jaw and the base of the tongue. The sublingual glands are located in the floor of your mouth. The submandibular and sublingual glands both release saliva under the tongue, producing the largest amount of saliva.

There are also many minor salivary glands inside your mouth, many of which are located near the lips, that produce limited amounts of saliva. The minor salivary glands are the glands that can be biopsied as part of the diagnostic evaluation for SjS.

"Mouth watering" is not just some copywriter's sales pitch. When you see and smell a delicious chocolate cake or a hamburger, your brain sends signals to your nerves, which tell these glands to produce saliva, and water flows into your mouth. Those with SjS have a malfunction in the process, a disturbance in both the major and minor glands. The dry mouth of SjS patients is the result of three dysfunctions:

- a decrease in the amount of saliva
- an alteration in the quality of the saliva
- changes in the cells that make the saliva

Most people have noticed how they lose saliva when they are stressed: The mouth goes dry. It could be that a stress state causes symptoms that mimic those of SjS. And chronic stress could make existing symptoms even worse. Given these possibilities, it is important for patients with autoimmune disorders to reduce the level of stress in their lives.

So the problem is not just limited to a reduction in the amount of saliva produced by these glands but also extends to its quality. These new pieces of understanding have helped frame and continue to direct research into promising new treatments for xerostomia.

Xerostomia is not limited to SjS patients. While it is a prominent component of SjS, it is also a feature in HIV infection, sarcoidosis, amyloidosis, and depression as well as the consequence of radiation therapy of the head and neck. It can also result from other disorders and medications, which makes diagnosis very tricky at times.

Testing for SjS: Salivary-Gland Biopsy

The most accepted test for SjS is the labial salivary-gland biopsy, but many patients are frightened at the prospect of having their lip sectioned and biopsied. The test is performed under local anesthetic and takes only a short time. It is possible that you will feel a numb sensation afterward.

The biopsy is taken from minor salivary glands of which there are many throughout the mouth, directly under the lips on the inside of the mouth. The incision is small and does not interfere with mouth function or speech. The scale for grading the results is from one to four, representing the number of white cells in that gland. A grade one result would not be enough to definitively diagnose SjS, but could be an indication of the disease. If the grade is four, the doctor will make a definite diagnosis of SjS upon finding the characteristic pattern of SjS under the microscope.

Symptoms of Dry Mouth

There are numerous oral symptoms associated with Sjögren's syndrome, many of which a dentist may notice during a checkup: multiple areas of decay, cracked teeth, an unusual loss of dental enamel at the base of the teeth, or periodontal infections. Often, the quality of the saliva in SjS patients changes from a somewhat clear, murky fluid to a thick, whitish mixture. A relatively common symptom is swollen parotid glands (located on the lower cheek area on both sides), much like mumps. Not all of these symptoms happen at one time, although any one of them could indicate to a patient or dentist the existence of SjS. But too often, symptoms occur intermittently, making a diagnosis difficult.

Today's dental schools include Sjögren's syndrome in their curricula, and young dentists are learning how to recognize it in its early stages. However, a dentist may not immediately correlate the symptoms with a

---

Medications That Can Cause Dry Mouth: Central Nervous System Agents

Medications are known to cause dry mouth. It is important to rule all of these out during the diagnostic period, so ask your doctor and pharmacist to check your list of medications for their drying effect.

Selective serotonin reuptake inhibitor antidepressants (Prozac, Paxil, Zoloft)

Antipsychotics (Risperdal, Clozaril)

Muscle relaxants (Baclofen, Flexeril)

Anti-Parkinsonian medications (Sinemet, Cogentin)

Chronic pain medications (Neurontin, Duragesic patches, Ultram)

Antihistamine allergy medications (Benadryl)

A British research study of fifty SjS patients found that twenty-three of the patients reported re-current or persistent salivary gland swelling with little relief. Researchers concluded that health professionals are failing to advise patients on symptom-reducing treatments. If you become de-pressed or feel isolated because of your symptoms, the time has come to join a SjS support group. Members of a support group can offer comfort and practical advice on dealing with the oppressive symptoms of SjS. The newsletter of the Sjögren's Syndrome Foundation lists contact persons in your area. Also, a telephone call to the foundation will help you find a group near you. See page 165 for web sites of the American and British SjS foundations.

disease like SjS if there are other causative factors that could cloud the di-agnosis. Dental training is improving in this regard, but often it is the rheumatologist who spots the disorder first and advises patients how to discuss it with their dentist.

Dental caries

If you are diagnosed with SjS by a rheumatologist, she will most likely inquire about recent dental work, any crowns you have needed, whether or not you need to drink water in order to swallow food or speak for a time, and whether lipstick sticks to your teeth. She will look under your tongue to assess whether the salivary pool is sufficient and check your tongue and mouth rim for sores and changes. If you wear dentures, you will be asked to remove them so the doctor can check the point at which the dentures meet the gum line.

Once you are diagnosed with SjS, you will immediately need to begin a regimen of preventive dental care that reaches beyond what your rheumatologist can provide. Your teeth will need to be checked often—at least every six months if possible—and you may need more frequent visits to the dental hygienist for professional cleanings and fluoride treatments. You will find it necessary to brush your teeth and floss between them more often during the day.

Tooth erosion is a serious problem for SjS patients who suffer from dry mouth, causing tooth decay (dental caries). And gum disease often follows tooth erosion. Your gums can become red and swollen and bleed easily. Your shrinking gum line will expose more of the tooth surface, which can decay. In severe cases your jawbone could become infected and your teeth could loosen as a result.

If your dentist thinks it necessary, you will receive a prescription for a mouth rinse called Peridex (Zila) or PerioGard (Colgate) in the United States and Peridex or Oro-Cleanse in Canada. These rinses are made with chlorhexidine, a substance that helps reduce inflammation and swelling of gums. He or she will advise you on mouth care and products that will keep you moist. Your dentist will also make you a set of fluoride gel carriers to be worn on your teeth with prescription fluoride for twenty minutes per day (much like a professional fluoride treatment) if recurrent decay is a problem for you. If you speak in public, you could be referred to a speech therapist to learn to preserve your abilities.

If you find that your dentist is unaware of the newer treatments for SjS-associated xerostomia, refer him to "Clinical Guidelines for Oral Treatment and Dental Caries Prevention in Patients with Chronic Dry Mouth" (2002) by Doctors Troy Daniels, Ava Wu, and Ernest Newbrun of the University of California at San Francisco (see Appendix). You and your dentist will both find it useful. Also, consider taking along a pamphlet on SjS from the Arthritis and Sjögren's Syndrome Foundation or your rheumatologist's office, or download a brief description from one of the SjS web sites listed in the Resources section at the back of this book.

Candidiasis

Saliva maintains the normal balance of the mouth's flora, protecting us from the overgrowth of organisms such as candida. For people with regular moisture in their mouth, candidiasis appears as white patches on the palate. SjS patients, however, present with red mucosa and a burning, painful tongue. There may also be little white spots at the back of the throat and soft palate. The complaints in all cases are the same: a burning, painful mouth and tongue with beefy red shiny patches or white lesions on the tongue and/or at the corners of the mouth. SjS patients usually show red, dry, cracked lesions at the side of the mouth rather than white ones. Often, those parts of the palate that are covered with dentures fall prey to this fungal infection, and the mucosa beneath the dentures appear red and inflamed.

Treatment for candidiasis must begin immediately and will require the use of topical medications for weeks or even months. Mouthwashes containing antifungal medications (like mycostatin) can be prescribed, or the use of solid antiyeast vaginal suppositories (such as nystatin troches) may be recommended. Topical antifungal ointment applied to the corners of the mouth often speeds the healing process. Some patients have also noted that increasing the amount of B-complex vitamins in their diet helps heal the lesions at the corners of the mouth.

Your physician or dentist may use the term *cheilosis,* meaning dryness and fissuring of the lips, to describe your condition. Cheilosis can result from vitamin deficiencies. The term *angular cheilitis* refers to this condition when it presents in the corners of the mouth. The good news is that it can be helped with medication and that treatment of oral candidiasis will help your symptoms. We have heard from dry-mouth sufferers that once the acute stage has been passed, eating unsweetened yogurt containing live culture and frequent brushing and flossing every day helps control the yeast. Other patients have reported success with a product that is available at health-food stores called Orithrush. It is a rinse that is used as a gargle.

Swollen glands

The parotid or submandibular glands of patients with SjS often become enlarged to varying degrees, sometimes causing pain. You feel and look like you did when you were a child with mumps. Sometimes the swellings will last for as long as a few weeks or months, and some sufferers have it on a continual basis.

To soothe the swelling and pain, apply hot compresses each day and then massage the glands. You can even do this in the shower by lathering up well and then massaging them gently. Or, when you are applying face cream, rub your fingers gently along the jaw line in front of and in back of your ear. Some massage therapists are particularly adept at face massages and can improve symptoms significantly. These techniques will not shrink the glands, but they will make them feel so much better.

TREATMENTS FOR DRY MOUTH

Your first line of defense at home with dry mouth is frequent brushing, flossing, and fluoride treatments. Your toothbrush should be soft, not hard or medium. Check the ingredients list on your toothpaste for sodium lauryl sulfate (SLS). SLS is a detergent, found in many toothpastes, that makes the paste foamy in your mouth. Unfortunately, it is believed to irritate the mucous layer of your mouth and to increase the likelihood of developing canker sores. Biotene, Rembrandt, and Dental Care for Sensitive

Teeth by Arm & Hammer, although a bit pricey, are three toothpastes without SLS.

Since water alone will not replace your saliva, dry-mouth gels and sprays can be efficient temporary moisturizers for your mouth. Try to avoid those containing alcohol. Artificial salivas are formulated to kill mouth bacteria, replace missing enzymes, and encourage the salivary glands to work. Items such as Salivart (Gebauer), Saliva Substitute (Rox-anne Laboratories), Optimoist (Colgate), Oral Balance (Laclede), and MouthKote (Parnell) are some of the products you will find in this cate-gory. In addition, BreathTech Plaque Fighter Mouth Spray (Omnii), Night-time Spray (Omnii), Tooth Towels (Comfy Concepts), Oragesic (Parnell), and Moi-Stir Swabs (Kingswood Laboratories) can prove helpful. Special dry-mouth gum (Biotene) will also help. There are also many specialized mouthwashes on the market, such as ACT (J&J), which contains fluoride, and Biotene (Laclede), which contains some of the enzymes ordinarily present in saliva.

Guaifenesin, a common ingredient in cough medications, is often used by SjS patients to thin the mucous secretions. For those who have success, it proves to be a splendid adjunct to other therapies. It can be found in Robitussin and in larger amounts, by prescription, as Humibid. Look for the formula for diabetics to reduce your sugar intake. Your phar-macist would be a good resource as to the various preparations, their po-tency, and possible side effects. It has been suggested that if the adult dose is hard to take, you may try the children's preparation. Some patients claim that it helps with some fibromyalgia symptoms as well, but this is a con-troversial subject within the medical community.

Water is, of course, extremely beneficial when attempting to soothe the symptoms of dry mouth, and you should always carry water with you to sip. You needn't drink a lot of water to help this condition: sips are what is required. In hot weather, suck on ice cubes, maybe even ice cubes made of lemonade (with artificial sweetener, of course). If your dryness leads to hoarseness and coughing, try a personal mist humidifier by your bed and on your desk.

There are many natural remedies for dry mouth as well. Slippery elm tea has been recommended by some as has deglycyrrhizinated licorice (DGL). DGL is the herb licorice (not the candy), and it is available in health-food stores. You can prepare a mouthwash with the powdered prod-uct and rinse, swish, and swallow, or alternatively, swallow the tablets and wash them down with water. This treatment has worked for some patients, especially those with canker sores. If you have vitamin E capsules in your house, try chewing on one before bed. It will coat your mouth while providing you with a necessary antioxidant. Similarly, adding olive oil to pasta and other dishes will moisturize your mouth as well as provide beneficial oils. And, in the same way, nut oils, such as walnut and hazelnut, will improve your diet while providing moisture and delicious taste. Another option is acupuncture, which has relieved the symptoms of xerostomia in some patients.

Use caution when drinking carbonated beverages; they decalcify teeth even if they are "diet," causing cavities. Avoid regular hard candy, gum, and drinks, but use sugar-free candy drops and gum. Always exercise caution, because even sugar-free candies contain citric acid, which is harmful to tooth enamel. Even a nice glass of wine is acidic to teeth and mucosa.

If All Else Fails . . . Try These

There are many people for whom saliva substitutes do not work. They are good candidates for the new medications called *secretagogues*. Presently there are two, available with a doctor's prescription: pilocarpine (Salagen), and cevimeline HCl (Evoxac). They are muscarinic agonists designed to stimulate residual salivary-gland activity. Both are in pill form, work systemically, and are aimed at improving the symptoms by increasing output from the salivary glands and tears from the lacrimal glands. They stimulate further secretion from glands that are still producing some, but not enough, saliva. Pilocarpine has been shown to stimulate salivary secretion and relieve symptoms of xerostomia in SjS patients. The recommended dose is 5 mg three to four times each day.

Cevimeline is a newer drug that has been shown to improve the symptoms of dry mouth and dry eye in patients with SjS. The dose is 30 mg three times a day although there have been reports of patients who get satisfaction with a lower dose, using one pill twice a day. Both drugs have been proven effective, although the cevimeline, which is taken fewer times a day, has a greater acceptance rate among users. Both drugs have side effects for some people, notably sweating (although somewhat less with cevimeline), and in some cases, nausea and gastrointestinal disturbances. However, patients for whom dry mouth is a serious problem adjust to the discomfort in order to get relief from the dryness.

These drugs, like all systemic medications, must be supervised by your physician. It is known that some chronic conditions preclude their use. Glaucoma, uncontrolled asthma, chronic bronchitis, obstructive pulmonary disease, and risk of cardiovascular diseases may mean that these drugs should be avoided. If either of these drugs is insufficient, your doctor may consider using immunomodulator agents, such as hydroxychloroquine, low-dose steroids, azathioprine, or methotrexate.

Sjögren's Syndrome and Your Ear, Nose, and Throat

Dry nose, throat, and bronchial tubes often bedevil patients with SjS. As well as causing discomfort, they can lead to infectious diseases that are difficult to cure. The disease can affect the exocrine glands in the upper respiratory tract as it does other target tissues. Dry nose can be helped with nasal gels applied at the opening, and dry throat can often be alleviated with a prescription form of guaifenesin, a common ingredient of over-the-counter cough medications. In both cases, they soften and loosen thickened and crusty mucous membranes. But what of the more troubling infectious diseases?

Sound familiar? Patients with SjS seem to succumb to more severe sinus symptoms than others. The lack of moisture results in paradoxical conditions. The mucous becomes more condensed, bulking up in the si-

---

Over the last ten years I have had increasingly close-together sinus "infections" whose primary symptom is intense pain—like a migraine—which responds well to a combination of antibiotics and prednisone. Rarely do I have drainage or even a stuffy nose, just terrible pain, the kind where bending over causes the sensation of someone hammering on my head. Nausea, vomiting, and inability to function at all or even stand up are common. My new ear, nose, and throat physician thinks my chronic sinus pain may be from one of three causes: chronic bacterial infection (maybe), chronic fungal infection (less likely, but can be tested), or, most likely, just plain old chronic inflammation of unknown etiology, just like what's happening already in many other parts of my body. If it's bacterial, endoscopic sinus surgery may help to improve drainage so I won't get the intense pain and get fewer infections. If it's fungal, antifungals will work. But if it's just plain inflammation, nothing will help except steroids, which are never a long-term solution.

—Claire

nus or throat; this thick secretion then puts out the welcome mat for invading viruses and ultimately for bacteria or fungi. And just as in Claire's case, the sinusitis and tracheitis can become chronic.

Sinusitis occurs when the mucous lining of the sinuses becomes inflamed. Anything that blocks the entry of air into the sinuses can result in inflammation: infections, allergies, polyps, or a deviated septum. SjS patients are particularly susceptible. When the sinus is affected, depending upon which one of the four is most inflamed, the symptoms may include pain in the upper jaw or cheek; tooth pain; pain, pressure, or swelling around the eye; and almost certainly, headache. These are signs of a latent sinus condition and should be addressed. Many people, especially those with chronic disease, try to ignore the symptoms, hoping they will go away on their own. However, avoidance of medical assessment and treatment can lead to irreversible changes in the sinus passageways.

Sometimes chronic sinus problems begin with a viral infection—a cold. There's nothing much that can be done with this beyond chicken soup and rest. But after seven to ten days, if there is still pain and drainage from your nose or throat, especially if it is yellow or green in color and not clear, you may have a bacterial infection that can be helped with antibiotics or nasal irrigation with topical antibiotics such as Bactroban. Since the sinus is clogged with tissue and because the blood supply to this area is limited, systemic antibiotics have difficulty reaching the infection in large enough amounts to banish the bacteria. But persist. Sometimes it can be helpful to have the ENT physician culture the sinus to see if the problem is a fungal infection, which would be treated with an antifungal medication rather than an antibiotic. Sometimes the same organism, such as a staphylococcus or streptococcus, will turn up repeatedly in the culture, which could suggest an underlying immunodeficiency disorder. This requires further investigation and may explain why some patients may get a systemic inflammatory/immune complex syndrome that follows the infection and does not respond to antibiotics but to anti-inflammatory or immunomodulator therapies. As a SjS sufferer, you may need to take antibiotics for longer than you expect. Do so, as removing a sinus infection is imperative. As with all antibiotics, provide your gastrointestinal tract with the appropriate bacteria by eating live-culture yogurt and enteric-coated probiotics two hours after a dose. Whichever you choose, keep up the sinus saline solutions, inhale steam as often as possible, and drink plenty of fluids to thin your nasal discharge.

And once your infection is gone, irrigate your sinus at least twice every day with saline solution. Salt water is a solvent; it cleans mucus from your nasal passages at the same time as it decongests your nose. Salt draws fluids out of the membranes. There are prepared compounds on the market that can be either dropped or sprayed, or you can prepare your own saline mixture. Whichever you choose, be sure to drip it into your nasal passages while you are bent over and stay that way for about a minute so that the solution will get right into the sinuses.

Saline Solution for Nasal Irrigation

> 1 quart or liter of warm water
> 2 to 3 teaspoons sea salt
> 1 teaspoon baking powder
> Bulb syringe, drop bottle, or WaterPik

Mix all the ingredients together and keep in a sterile jar in the refrigerator for no longer than one week. With a bulb syringe, drop bottle, or Water-Pik, stand over the sink and aim the liquid toward the back of your head, not the top, allowing some of it to drip into and out of your mouth. Clean the salt container carefully, in the dishwasher or with boiling water, each day. Use every day.

A product containing the natural anti-inflammatory substance yerba santa can also help and is available for irrigation and spray: Pretz Spray and Pretz Irrigation by Parnell (1-800-457-4276).

CAN YOU PREVENT SINUS INVOLVEMENT?

Humidity in your bedroom will help; sinus irrigation or moisture sprays will also help. Be certain that your humidifier is checked and cleaned often so that fungi don't become resident and then airborne. Check the status of your allergies; they can lead to sinus problems. And if you are a swimmer, avoid forcing pool water up your nose when diving. The chlorine in the pool can exacerbate inflammation in your sinus, and if you are fortunate enough to find a pool that is cleaned with ozone instead of chlorine, you will find your symptoms will be fewer. And finally, if your difficulty does not yield, surgery can be an effective option.

Some patients have found that an asthma-prevention medicine (Singulair), which inhibits the leukotriene inflammation pathway, taken orally at night can prevent sinus infections. Some patients will use this just during "high-risk periods" in the winter or flu season. The benefit of taking this drug is a reduction in the amount of antibiotics taken for infections, which is indeed a help. Also, some patients may benefit from using doxycycline, a tetracycline antibiotic that inhibits the metalloproteinase inflammatory pathway and thus has anti-inflammatory properties. It can serve to prevent the "typical" sinus infections and can be used for two-week- to several-month-long intervals as needed. Some allergists recommend using doxy-cycline a few days before and post airplane travel if the patient's pattern has been to contract frequent sinus or upper respiratory infections following airplane travel.

Another therapy, sometimes recommended by sinus specialists, is a steroid nasal spray used each day as a prophylactic to avoid inflammation in the sinus passages.

THYROID INVOLVEMENT

The thyroid gland can also become involved with an autoimmune attack. If low thyroid function (hypothyroidism) develops, it will contribute to the dryness and fatigue. Thyroid involvement is not an uncommon find-ing in SjS patients and can slowly sneak up on you if you are not thinking about it. Fortunately, the problem can be fairly easily detected by a blood test called *thyroid-stimulating hormone* (TSH), and the autoimmune process can be confirmed with the presence of thyroid peroxidase antibod-ies. Occasionally, the thyroid will be found to be overactive, and diseases such as Grave's disease and Hashimoto's thyroiditis (an autoimmune con-dition) may be diagnosed and require additional treatment. In hypo-thyroidism, supplemental thryoid medications are given and the dose regulated to not oversuppress the TSH, which could result in osteoporosis.

CHAPTER 6

Extraglandular Involvement

WHILE MODERATING A PANEL AT THE SJÖGREN'S Syndrome Foundation Seminar in Atlanta (April 2002), a rheumatologist surprised his audience when he warned, "If your ophthalmologist diagnosed your disease, you don't have it! Those people who have not seen a rheumatologist make a mistake. It's a complete syndrome, not an isolated area, not all dry eyes and dry mouth are Sjögren's syndrome. This is a multisystem disorder."

So far we have discussed the effect on the exocrine or moisture-producing glands. Now we will look at nonexocrine disease. Primary Sjögren's syndrome (SjS) can cause disturbance of the gastrointestinal tract,

I have problems with digestion. Food seems to just sit in my stomach, and I have what I think is heartburn. Sometimes I have impossible constipation, which makes me uncomfortable. But mostly I suffer with nausea, bloating, tendernesss, and gas—sort of like my stomach is going to explode. I have been told that it is a motility problem, and the other day I was told that it is also a problem with my nervous system. Is this part of Sjögren's syndrome?

—Janet

kidneys, circulation, nervous system, muscles, joints, skin, lungs, vagina, bladder, bone marrow, and lymph glands.

Perhaps you have had feelings of food "sticking" in your esophagus. Or you have pain in your stomach, bloating, indigestion, nausea, and trouble with constipation or difficulty passing a stool. Could this be SjS? Yes, anywhere along the tract—esophagus, stomach, small and large intestine, colon—or off the tract—pancreas and liver—SjS can be the culprit.

Digestive Disorders

It certainly could be a part of the systemic nature of the disorder, but it could also be related to diet, medications, stress, or emotional factors. Also, if you have secondary SjS, your digestive difficulties could be related to another autoimmune disease, such as scleroderma or lupus. Unfortunately, there is not much in the literature about these symptoms. Few researchers have made this their area of investigation; much of the treatment tends to be focused on symptom relief rather than an understanding of the basic cause. A lot of what is known and practiced by specialists is based on the doctor's clinical experience; there is no national or international database for these disorders.

DYSPHAGIA

Patients with SjS complain of *dysphagia* or difficulty in swallowing due to dryness of the pharynx and esophagus or abnormal esophageal motility. Nausea and epigastric pain are common. This is largely due to the decrease in the saliva necessary to coat food and allow it to slip down the esophagus smoothly. Abnormal esophageal motility is often diagnosed when the muscles of the esophagus, wanting to mulch the food and pass it to the stomach, are weak from poor coordination.

HEARTBURN

Heartburn in SjS is common because the esophagus muscles are sluggish; acid is regurgitated into the esophagus, causing inflammation and pain. Stomach acid is ordinarily blocked from backing up into the esophagus by the lower esophageal sphincter, a circular band of muscles at the lower end of the esophagus that normally remain closed except during swallowing. If the sphincter becomes weakened, stomach acid can reflux up and burn the lower esophagus. This is more severe in SjS and, if left too long, will lead to scarring and further narrowing of the passage or even to a more serious condition, Barrett's esophagus. Symptoms of pain and burning in the esophagus require attention.

Look for a gastrointestinal specialist (gastroenterologist) who has some understanding of autoimmune disorders to assess your condition. He or she will likely perform an upper endoscopy to determine the cause and treatment of this disturbance in your digestive process. The investigation is brief and performed under mild anesthetic. It will locate the injury, and a biopsy will analyze the health of the tissue. Early diagnosis and treatment can forestall further erosion and painful symptoms.

GASTROESOPHAGEAL REFLUX DISEASE

Gastroesophageal reflux disease (GERD) is the term applied to the symptoms or tissue damage caused by reflux of the stomach's contents (usually acidic) into the esophagus. Heartburn, nausea, and discomfort may indicate GERD. It can be treated medically and must be supervised by your rheumatologist or GI specialist. Self-medication is not advised in these circumstances. It's tempting to try heavily advertised medications such as Zantac or Pepcid and avoid yet another doctor's appointment, but it is probably shortsighted. This is a condition that can be helped, but it needs to be supervised medically and may require stronger medications used for longer periods than those for peptic ulcer disease in the average person.

And bear in mind that the medications that are used by patients with SjS are sometimes worse than the condition for which they were prescribed. The chemical and physical properties of the drug, the formulation, and the size and shape of the tablet or capsule can play a role in the injury of the GI tract. Medications that are taken with inadequate liquid may become sticky as they dissolve and delay the transit time of the drug. They may become lodged in the esophagus and injure the lining. Tablets should always be taken with a full glass of liquid.

There are things you can do to feel better. To support your healing, drink plenty of water with your meals. Take small bites and chew food thoroughly. Eat small meals throughout the day rather than large meals at breakfast, lunch, and dinner. Have your last small meal at least two hours before bed. Remember that there is a tendency to regurgitate esophageal contents when lying down. You may prop your bed's head up so that food will move down rather than back up. There are special bed supports available at medical supply stores, but a few thick blocks laid under the head of the mattress or bed legs will often do the trick.

STOMACH INFLAMMATION

Perhaps you suffer with symptoms of nausea or fullness in the upper abdomen and a burning in your midsection. Patients with these symptoms often have chronic inflammation of the stomach. The stomach may not empty normally, much as diabetics develop a condition called *gastroparesis,* a neurological paralysis of the muscular coat of the stomach. It is believed that neurotransmitters may play a role. Then again, an autoantibody, the parietal cell antibody, can inhibit production of much-needed hydrochloric acid. Acid is needed for optimal food digestion. Medications for this condition do exist. Again decide on your treatment in concert with your physician. Some patients report using ginger to successfully manage nausea. Ginger candies are tempting, but since they are made with sugar you might try instead grated ginger over fruit salad, lots of ginger in stir-fry dinners, and tiny slivers of ginger over grilled fish.

Still other patients regularly supplement their meals with enteric-coated digestive enzymes, also sold as *probiotics.* These are gelcaps, tablets, or powder that contain organisms that can be lost from the GI tract, especially when you are taking antibiotics. Digestive enzymes or probiotics are sold in health-food stores and should be stored in a refrigerated case in the store and in your refrigerator or freezer at home. When shopping, search for those that can withstand the acid in your stomach, labeled "enteric coated."

PANCREATIC COMPLAINTS

The pancreas can be affected in SjS patients. You may feel a dull pain around the stomach (epigastric) where the pancreas is located, and sometimes there is radiation of the pain to the back. Abnormalities can usually be seen in blood tests (elevated pancreatic amylase or lipase). Again, inflammation is the hallmark. Since the pancreas makes enzymes that are important to digestion, the symptoms may be those of poor digestion or even malabsorption when important nutrients are not absorbed from the intestine. Treatment may be needed if the totality of the symptoms warrants. Trying pancreatic enzymes for limited periods could be enough.

LIVER COMPLAINTS

The liver may be involved in the symptoms as well. This organ is located in the right upper abdomen. Pain from inflammation or associated autoimmune hepatitis antibodies, which are directed at various proteins within the liver cells, can be an outcome of Sjögren's syndrome. Since the liver plays such an important role in clearing toxins from the body, its malfunction can produce symptoms of fatigue and general malaise. Routine blood tests can detect the liver damage, and specialized autoantibodies can further define the process. Usually this is a minor issue in SjS, and specific treatment is not generally prescribed. Sometimes hydroxychloroquine (Plaquenil), a medication given most often for associated arthritis, can improve the lab studies and symptoms.

BLOATING AND CONSTIPATION

The causes of bloating and constipation in SjS patients are uncertain, possibly a combination of infiltration of lymphocytes and neuropathy that causes dysmotility. Since the production of moist substances declines from so many other glands and organs, one can expect that the stool would be less lubricated and lose more fluid because of the slower transit time in the GI tract. Thus the stool will become harder and more difficult to pass.

Self-treatment is *not* the route to wellness. You should have your doctor prescribe laxatives or guide you to over-the-counter treatments for the long term. Take the time to discuss all your symptoms with your doctor. Make sure to have a list of the daily medications you take when designing a regimen for problems of the intestine and colon. It's tempting to self-prescribe, particularly when over-the-counter medications are advertised so heavily and are readily available. It is possible that some of the laxatives will interact with the other drugs you may be taking. This is a long-term management problem and one that needs thought and planning. Better have a regimen tailor-made to fit you!

After your physician has ruled out the possibility of serious consequences from your symptoms, you may be left with some decision making of your own. Occasional constipation happens to everyone. The everyday recommendation to eat more fiber, drink more fluids, and exercise more often just won't work if your gastric distress is caused by dysmotility or inflammation from SjS. You need to understand that laxatives work in different ways, so choose from among them carefully, after a discussion with your doctor.

Oral Laxatives

Oral laxatives fall into five categories: bulk forming, hyperosmotic, stimulant, lubricant, and stool softeners. In each category there are combinations designed to evacuate the stool more easily. It is probably wise to avoid laxatives that are a combination of two or more categories. One drug at a time is more reliable.

Bulk-forming laxatives: These absorb liquid from the intestines and swell to form a soft bulky stool. They are not digested. These are gentle but, depending upon the severity of the symptoms, may not be effective for SjS patients.

- Active ingredient: methylcellulose, psyllium, bran, polycarbophil
- Commonly used brand names: Citrucel, Metamucil, FiberCon caplets, Mylanta Natural Fiber, Pro-Lax, Serutan

Hyperosmotic laxatives: These draw water from surrounding tissues into the bowel. They increase the action of the bowel and provide a soft stool for easier passage. There are three types of hyperosmotics: saline or "salts," lactulose, and polymer.

- *Saline:* Draw water into bowel, can be harsh.
  - Active ingredient: magnesium citrate, magnesium hydroxide, sodium phosphate, magnesium sulfate heptahydrate.
  - Commonly used brand names: Citroma, Fleet Phospho-soda, Epsom salts, Phillips' chewable and concentrated Milk of Magnesia
- *Lactulose:* A sugar that works more slowly than saline. Some people react strongly.
  - Active ingredient: lactulose
  - Commonly used brand names (available by prescription only): Constilac, Constulose, Heptalac, Portalac

- *Polymer:* Causes water to be held in the stool and increases the number of bowel movements.
  - Active ingredient: polyethylene glycol
  - Commonly used brand name (available by prescription only): Miralax

Stimulant laxatives: These encourage bowel movements by increasing muscle contractions of the intestinal wall causing the stool to move through the tract. Since they have potential side effects, it is important to discuss their use with your physician.

- Active ingredients: bisacodyl, cascara sagrada, castor oil, senna, sennosides (Patients report that senna, sennosides, and bisacodyl are gentle.)
- Commonly used brand names: Correctol, Dacodyl, Dulcolax, Ex-Lax, Fleet Stimulant Laxative, Nature's Remedy, Senokot, Senolax

Lubricant laxatives: These coat the stool as well as the tract lining with a waterproofing and therefore keep moisture in the stool. Since SjS patients suffer from a lack of moisture, this method may not be effective.

- Active ingredient: mineral oil
- Commonly used brand name: mineral oil

Stool softeners: These help the patient evacuate the stool by helping liquid mix through the dry matter. Because of the shortage of moisture in an SjS patient, these may not be sufficient for an effective clearing of the bowel but may be useful in combination with a gentle stimulant or hyperosmotic laxative.

- Active ingredient: docusate sodium, docusate calcium
- Commonly used brand names: Colace, Doxidan, Correctol Stool Softener, Fleet Soflax Gelcaps, Sulfolax, Surfak

Digestion Aids

Sometimes, your stomach needs a rest. A small percentage of SjS patients suffer from a condition known as *gastroparesis,* or a slowing down of the stomach's emptying. The symptoms are difficult: a feeling of fullness, bloating, and pain, and is usually accompanied by constipation and

GERD. When this happens, it might be a good idea to give the stomach a rest by following some simple rules at mealtimes:

- Eat slowly and chew thoroughly.
- Try to eat in relaxing circumstances, perhaps with easygoing friends and family. Avoid stressful events such as the evening news as you eat.
- Try for frequent small meals rather than three big ones.
- Remember that the more liquid your food is, the faster it will pass through. You may want to have a liquid meal occasionally.
- Purée your meats with broth to render them more digestible.
- Mix baby food with juice or broth as a transitional food, halfway between a solid and a liquid.
- Use a juicer to concoct fresh fruit and vegetable drinks daily. (You get a wider assortment of enzymes and whole-food nurients in this way.)
- Cooked food is easier on your GI tract than raw food, so go for applesauce, yogurt, soy milk, thick juices, puréed soups, and runny oatmeal.
- Eat low-fat, high-fiber foods for easier digestion.
- Don't sit still after eating. Moving around usually helps digestion.

Food Allergies

Food allergies have been suspected as triggers of SjS. Foods such as dairy products, wheat, corn, eggs, and others can be the invisible components of everyday life that cause our symptoms and discomfort. One of the most common is celiac disease. Nearly 1 in 150 Americans suffers from celiac disease. Surprisingly, most people think it is a rare condition. In the autoimmune population, it is relatively common. Celiac disease, an autoimmune disorder, is a digestive disease that damages the small intestine and interferes with the absorption of nutrients, particularly vitamin B_{12}. People who have celiac disease cannot tolerate gluten, a protein found in wheat, rye, barley, and possibly oats. Gluten is the protein that gives bread its texture, makes a pizza crust chewy, and allows a cake to rise and set. When people with celiac disease eat foods containing gluten, their immune system responds by damaging the small intestine, specifically the tiny fingerlike protrusions, called *villi*, on the lining of the small intestine. In many cases the symptoms are not typical of digestive problems.

Symptoms such as recurring abdominal bloating and pain, chronic diarrhea, weight loss, pale and foul-smelling stool, unexplained anemia, gas, bone and joint pain, muscle cramps, fatigue, and a painful skin rash called *dermatitis herpetiformis* can be signs of celiac disease. They can also be signs of SjS. Of clinical interest is the fact that the autoimmune-disease susceptibility gene, HLA–DR3, is common to both disorders.

There are tests for celiac disease. Researchers have discovered that people with celiac disease have higher than normal levels of certain antibodies in their blood. These antibodies swoop into the bloodstream to react against the threat of gluten. Your blood can be tested for antibodies such as antigliadin, antiendomysium, and transglutamate. A gluten-free diet sounds austere; in reality it is quite manageable and, if your symptoms are caused by celiac disease, rewarding. You will have more energy, eliminate some symptoms, and achieve a level of health you didn't know was possible.

Components in your foods other than gluten could also be responsible for your symptoms. An "elimination diet" will identify food allergies by eliminating specific foods or groups of foods from the diet one at a time. You eliminate all the suspected foods for two weeks, then begin to add each food back until one or more of them triggers symptoms. This does not mean you can never eat these foods again! Often when the "flare" is resolved you can eat moderate amounts of the problem foods without the symptoms. Eliminating the trigger foods when a "flare" occurs will often help resolve the problem more quickly.

Urinary-System Disorders

Irritable bladder syndrome, which is a painful disorder of the urinary bladder characterized by urgency, frequency, pain, and a need to urinate during the night, without infection occurs often in SjS. The recurrent theme of lymphocyte infiltration is implicated. It is difficult to diagnose with certainty because the biopsies of the bladder may do more harm in the long run. Usually, just understanding that this is yet another feature of the disease is reassuring. It is often possible to discontinue the antibiotics that are often prescribed for these symptoms. Occasionally, in severe cases, the anti-inflammatory agent DMSO is instilled into the bladder by a urologist. Very occasionally the kidneys are affected with various conditions, including renal tubular acidosis, interstitial nephritis, and renal stones.

Pulmonary-System Disorders

When there is involvement of the pulmonary system—the lungs and tra-chea—there will be complaints of chronic hoarseness, tickling in the throat, and an almost constant need to clear the throat. There is a chronic, nonproductive cough mimicking asthmatic bronchitis, chronic bronchitis, or even asthma. There could be a feeling of shortness of breath (dyspnea), which may trigger doctors to advise their patients to lose weight or exercise more. To a rheumatologist, these symptoms suggest possible inflammation in the pulmonary system. Dyspnea is subtle and not usually severe. Pa-tients often consider it unimportant and not critical enough to mention to a rheumatologist. It takes considerable questioning to uncover symptoms like these. They could mean that there is a possible dryness of tracheo-bronchial mucosa with a secondary low-grade infection caused by the dry-ness and inadequate clearance of the infective agents by the immune system. It could be a reaction to a medication; check with your doctor. It could mean infiltration of lymphocytes anywhere in the system. Lymphocytes can infiltrate different areas of the pulmonary system. Depending upon where they have accumulated, tests can be initiated that will direct attention to the correct spot, and these results, in turn, will dictate treatment options.

For example, if lymphocytic infiltrates occur in the *parenchyma* (sup-portive tissue) of the lung, the interstitial infiltrates could be seen on a chest X-ray if severe or on a high-resolution chest CT scan if mild or early in development. Occasionally the most sensitive test will be a formal pulmonary-function test, which must include diffusion capacity to mea-sure the actual ability of oxygen to perfuse from the air breathed in and transported into the bloodstream. Often the diffusion capacity will be de-creased. This strongly suggests that cellular infiltrate or scarring has oc-curred in the interstitium, leading to a diagnosis of interstitial lung disease. Only a lung biopsy will confirm the diagnosis and reveal what the intersti-tial process is, whether a fibrosis or cellular infiltrate. A cellular infiltrate process is highly reversible if treated with immune modulators such as prednisone. Fibrosis is probably irreversible with currently available agents, although some in clinical development hold the promise of treating and reversing the fibrosis.

If the chest X-ray or other imaging study has revealed a *hilar adenopa-*

thy (swelling of the lymph glands at the part of the organ where the vessels enter and leave), *mediastinal adenopathy* (swelling of the lymph nodes in the chest area), or nodules in the lung, the physician will suspect a pseudolymphoma or lymphoma. A lung biopsy will need to be performed in order to confirm the diagnosis. If free fluid appears to be forming between the lung and the interpleural space, it is generally in the presence of secondary SjS, most commonly lupus. SjS patients display an anomoly in that when these effusions occur they can contain lymphocytes and even the autoantibodies SSA/SSB that are identified with SjS.

All that said, however, the prognosis for the successful treatment of such conditions is good. Even the lymphomas, treated with specialized lymphoma protocols, have a high success rate.

It is important, then, to have diagnostic consultation with a lung specialist when any of the symptoms of coughing, wheezing, dryness, and infection become troublesome. The tests will rule out complications. If the symptoms are mild and not too intrusive, you can institute strategies for moistening the breathing passages. An air washer or steamer will provide relief; removal of drying medications (see page 66) will help. The breathing of steamy hot air several times a day will make life easier. Bronchial spasms can be managed with the occasional use of bronchodilators, and when local mucosa are inflamed, steroid inhalers will contain the inflammation. Anecdotal evidence supports the use of Singulair, a leukotriene inhibitor approved for use with asthma, to be effective in the prevention of infection. Make sure that you treat infections quickly and do everything you can to remain infection-free.

When interstitial lung disease becomes problematic, the area can be tapped to remove fluid; usually NSAIDs or steroids will be the treatment of choice. A diagnosis of SjS along with the other complications provides a window into the process that is contributing to the symptoms. This is important. It means that simple interventions such as NSAIDs and steroids will be the treatments of choice.

Circulatory-System Disorders

It is very uncommon for a person with SjS to present with cardiac symptoms; however, it happens. This phenomenon is probably underinvestigated by researchers and certainly is rarely considered by clinicians. Only a few studies appear in the literature that look at types of heart involvement and incidence.

Often, if a patient with heart symptoms seeks counsel from a cardiologist or internist, the symptoms of dry eyes and mouth are not considered clinically significant, and the possibility of SjS is rarely addressed.

Your symptoms may indicate that you should have an electrocardiogram. While highly unusual, when SjS is present, there could be heart involvement resulting from the presence of fluid caused by inflammation in the space between the heart and the protective lining of the pericardial sac. This is called *asymptomatic pericarditis.* Another condition uncovered with an electrocardiogram is increased pulmonary artery pressure, which you would experience as increased and severe shortness of breath. The test for this usually requires a right-heart catheterization.

If you notice that your legs are swelling or getting puffy, a trip to the doctor is warranted. This and increased heart rate are possible with inflammatory disorders and should be considered as diagnostic tools for heart disease.

The prognosis for any of these conditions is good, especially if linked to SjS and treated early. Such possibilities are not as bad as they sound. Usually, once SjS is seen as a cofactor in any of these conditions, treatments to reduce inflammation can make a positive difference in the outcome.

Musculoskeletal-System Disorders

Half of all patients with primary SjS have episodes of arthritis sometime during their disease. For some it is chronic. You may experience joint pains that travel as a result of swelling of the knee or shoulder, chronic arthritis of several joints—notably those of the fingers—and a feeling of stiffness on rising in the morning. All of these are signs of inflammation. Distinct from the arthritis of rheumatoid arthritis, this type does not cause erosions of bone. Perhaps you have experienced the problem, but the episodes have resolved, so you have not brought them to your doctor's attention. Perhaps you have already consulted an orthopedic surgeon, even undergone arthroscopy without a specific diagnosis, and upon review of the pathology report there was mention of nonspecific inflammation or a lymphocytic infiltrate. In spite of this, and the fact that the problem was not resolved as you would have liked, the possibility of SjS was not considered. But it is a consideration.

Arthralgia, mild inflammation of the joints, and arthritis, which is a more severe form of the same thing, present pain and discomfort that require a physician's visit for relief. This is not the arthritis of rheumatoid arthritis (RA). SjS arthritis is very different and should not be confused with RA. RA is a very inflammatory arthritis usually causing detectable *synovitis* (inflammation of a synovial membrane, especially that of a joint), which can be observed by examining the knuckles of the hands and toes. It is symmetrical. SjS arthritis is generally more of an arthralgia with symptoms of inflammation in which the synovitis is not detectable on examination. The joints affected most often are the small joints of the hands, and it is more asymmetric. Also larger joints, such as the shoulders and knees, can be involved. In general it is less inflammatory than RA and thus responds to milder and lower doses of medications.

Fortunately, SjS arthritis is a condition that can be managed by both the patient and the doctor. The first question is, is it severe or mild? A physical examination will quickly reveal the answer. If the doctor discovers residual deformity of a joint or bulges in the joint, she will diagnose arthritis. If not, it is arthralgia. Any deformity or bump is a residue of the inflammation that happened earlier. Pain is secondary to inflammation, unless there has been structural damage to joints or tendons, in which case the pain is secondary to mechanical problems.

Here is where the doctor plays a role. Since SjS arthritis is similar to rheumatoid arthritis and the arthritis of lupus, she will prescribe nonsteroidal anti-inflammatories, such as ibuprofen, or the newer Cox-2 inhibitors (Celebrex or Vioxx) or hydroxychloroquine (Plaquenil) or methotrexate (Methotrex). Hydroxychloroquine is commonly used in the arthritis of lupus, and NSAIDs, low-dose prednisone and methotrexate are still the most common medications used to treat rheumatoid arthritis. Anecdotally it has been reported that the arthralgia/arthritis of SjS responds to the asthma medication Singulair, which inhibits a pathway of inflammation called *leukotrienes.*

And the patient can begin using soothing self-help remedies like heat, hot-wax baths, and warm-water hand baths with gentle range-of-motion exercises. Water exercise is a supportive, helpful way to reduce pain and increase range of motion.

Skin Disorders

About one third of those with SjS suffer from a discoloration of feet and hands called *Raynaud's disease.* The extremities feel very cold and look distinctly misshapen. Raynaud's syndrome is a vascular spasm of the small vessels, usually restricted to the hands and feet but sometimes appearing in the small vessels leading to other organs. It is rare and more common to find these complications in scleroderma or lupus; however, it is also possible with SjS.

Occasionally Raynaud's disease will have been present since the teen years. It is rarely seen in childhood. The "classic" presentation of Raynaud's disease is three-color changes of the digits: white, which indicates decreased blood flow; blue, which shows decreased oxygen secondary to decreased blood flow; and red, which indicates increased blood perfusion when the vessel opens up. The cause is irritability and spasm of the small blood vessels. If the condition becomes severe, small ulcers will develop at the tips of the fingers or toes because of insufficient blood and nutrients.

Anything that will increase blood circulation will help. Keep your hands and feet as warm as possible by using warm paraffin baths and heat; decrease stress; practice biofeedback, yoga, or qi gong, all of which increase circulation and provide mild relief. Some medications may be called for. For example, calcium channel blockers, which are used for high blood pressure treatment, may help prevent the spasm. If your blood pressure is normal this medicine could make it abnormally low and cause dizziness and fatigue.

There can be many skin changes with SjS, anything from dry, itchy skin to small, deep red-purple spots about the size of a dime that are usually on your legs or arms. The most likely complication is dry skin; the least likely, the purpura or purple spots. Those who have dry skin need to avoid water, particularly hot water. The best way to manage this annoying condition is to use a body scrub in the shower or bath to remove the dry dead cells from the surface, leave your body only slightly toweled off, and immediately apply a body moisturizer. Rich, thick creams rather than lotions are best. Applied on a thick dead cell layer, even the best creams will yield little benefit. Keeping skin moist is essential if you suffer from dry skin.

The purple spots are signs of vasculitis of the very small blood vessels and often present no problem unless they are many and unsightly. Prognosis for small-vessel vasculitis affecting the skin is excellent. Usually it is resolved through the normal body's repair mechanism. If it is diagnosed early in the process, the effects can be reversed. If you notice any of these symptoms, it would be wise to bring them to your doctor's attention early.

Possible treatments are topical steroids for rashes and ingested steroids for most types of vasculitis, but if steroids are needed for longer periods of time, then steroid-sparing agents such as azathioprine or methotrexate are used. If this is the case, consult a dermatologist for suggestions or discuss with your rheumatologist the possibility of using mild steroid-containing creams or a stronger nonsteroidal immunomodular cream approved for atopic dermatitis (Protopic Ointment Fujisawa). This ointment comes in two strengths, 0.03% or 0.1%, and does not thin the skin like topical steroids can. The treatment will be cosmetic rather than curative, but in many cases, this can give a sufferer overall peace of mind.

Nervous-System Disorders

Both the peripheral nervous system, which serves the arms and legs, and the central nervous system, which serves the brain and spinal cord, can be compromised with SjS. Such conditions are not readily diagnosed.

Peripheral neuropathy may appear after other symptoms of SjS appear or, even more disconcerting, may precede them. The onset can be slow and insidious. It can attack single nerves that dysfunction and become numb, resulting in a condition called *mononeuritis multiplex*. This is most commonly found in the peroneal nerve of the foot, exhibited as a condition known as "foot drop." It can also affect multiple nerves. Peripheral neuropathy can be troubling because the burning of the nerve endings is usually in the feet and hands, places where dexterity, movement, and pressure are needed for everyday activities. If it is diagnosed early, it may be reversed. If later, treatment tends to be palliative.

Diagnosis is done by a neurologist, who will look for evidence of sensory and motor malfunction using EMG (electromyography) and nerve-conduction studies to objectively assess the status of the nerve fibers in the affected area. At times, these tests may be normal, especially in cases of small-fiber neuropathy. Further testing, perhaps a skin biopsy along the affected nerve, is required. But this presupposes an awareness on the part of the doctor and patient that SjS can contribute to peripheral neuropathy. Furthermore, if there are no other signs of SjS, it is a particularly challenging task to diagnose. The ideal arrangement would be to have an informed patient work with a team of specialists, including a rheumatologist and a neurologist.

Autonomic neuropathy is another form of peripheral neuropathy. In this condition, the neuropathy is directed to the autonomic nervous system, that part of the nervous system over which we have little control. The autonomic nervous system, which activates our stomach muscles, helps us breathe, and circulates our blood, can malfunction with SjS. Autonomic neuropathy has vague, difficult-to-diagnose symptoms that cause a patient to doubt her own illness. Light-headedness, dizziness, fatigue when active, and various gastrointestinal disorders, like bloating and constipation, could signify a neuropathy of the autonomic nervous system. It is probably fairly common, but the vague symptoms are puzzling and often ignored. Autonomic neuropathy can affect blood pressure. Normally, pulse rates rise when a person goes from a prone to a standing position so that normal blood pressure is maintained. In autonomic neuropathy, because of a condition called *orthostatic hypotension*, the pulse will not rise and blood pressure will drop. There are other symptoms as well: absence of sweating, sluggish response of the pupil of the eye (Adie's syndrome), temperature dysregulation, vasospasm (a bumplike reaction on the skin when pressure is applied), and dysmotility of the GI tract, resulting in severe constipation and a type of pseudo-obstruction syndrome.

Difficult to diagnose and perhaps even more difficult to treat, neuropathies present a problem for both patient and physician. The patient truly feels unwell but has only vague symptoms that are difficult to describe. The physician must rely on clinical experience and judgment, as there are few objective tests.

There are treatments for peripheral neuropathies. However, they are not effective for long-term use. If the condition is diagnosed early, it may be reversed. One of the strategies for early reversal is the regular infusion of intravenous immunoglobulin (IVIG), which has been found to be an effective treatment when the neuropathy is discovered early in its development. Medicinal treatments can be helpful in sorting through the possible causes of the dysfunctions, but the side effects of the treatments can be unpleasant. Most of the treatments are steroid-based and come with the damaging side effects of all steroids. The first challenge is to decide whether there is inflammation at work. At times, if the neuropathies have been present for a long time, scar tissue will form. Scar tissue is irreversible. If the symptoms are severe and there is a degree of inflammatory or immune-mediated signs as compared with an accumulation of scar tissue in the affected nerves, the physician may decide that a short course of steroids could be effective, both as a diagnosis and as beginning treatment. These will shortly be discontinued and followed with steroid-sparing agents (DMARDs) for ongoing treatment.

Home remedies for neuropathies are many. If the physician feels that medical interventions will do little to relieve the symptoms, treatment tends to be palliative. Physical therapy, good nutrition with added antioxidants, and medications are ways of managing the pain. High-dose vitamin E has been shown to be effective in neuropathies. A daily intake of 2,000 IU of vitamin E can help with symptoms.

An excellent resource for those seeking information on neuropathies is the Neuropathy Association, based in New York City. Their newsletter, *Neuropathy News,* and the member-service chat line on their web site are helpful.

Both the cranial nerve and the central nervous system may be affected by SjS. These conditions are very rare and are treatable. Patients with SjS sometimes complain of "brain fog," changes in cognitive function: memory loss, loss of attention, and difficulty concentrating. SjS can have an effect on the cognitive processes of the nervous system. If you suffer from any of these functional changes, remind your physician that you have SjS; it is important for diagnosis. In SjS the nerve is being attacked by inflammatory cells, or the blood vessel that feeds the nerve is being attacked. This results in decreased blood flow and nutrients which damage the nerves as a secondary effect. As it is with peripheral neuropathies, the prognosis is usually good with early diagnosis and treatment.

It is clear that extraglandular involvement can have troubling and far-reaching effects in SjS. Once diagnosed, however, there are treatment options available. Including SjS in your medical history and being aware of the possibilities of extraglandular complications will help both patient and doctor achieve successful interventions and prevent further illness.

CHAPTER 7

Pain and Fatigue

Pain

Manhattan-born Dahlia reflects the experience of the majority of SjS patients when she describes her pain as "unbearable." She is joined by all of those who feel the muscle, joint, and nerve pain of this disorder and others. Chronic pain, and by this we mean unrelenting pain for longer than six months, afflicts from 30 to 50 million Americans. At one time or another, almost everyone with Sjögren's syndrome (SjS) experiences debili-

I was pregnant with my third child when the pain started. I blamed my pregnancy, but when it continued after my daughter's birth I began to get concerned. The muscle pain and fatigue were trying my patience. There were times when I thought I would not be able to look after the children; the pain was unbearable and my tiredness made me cranky. Luckily, my gynecologist referred me to a rheumatologist who did blood tests and diagnosed Sjögren's syndrome. I have been using a combination of massage, warm baths, and medications, and can finally enjoy being with the children, but it was touch and go there for a while.

—Dahlia

tating pain, sometimes for short but often for long periods. And because society teaches us that people who try to make sense of their pain are complainers, wimps, or whiners, our first inclination when pain hits is to depreciate it. A broken leg has earned its pain; a seemingly well person with pain is dubbed a whiner. But pain is a signal. It needs early intervention and will worsen if it continues untreated. Chronic pain can last long after normal healing and treatment should have removed it.

"We All Have Some Pain—Get Used to It!"

How often have you heard that? And, perhaps more important, how often have you said that to yourself? Society sanctions a self-critical attitude toward pain, but nature dictates the opposite: Recognize it, authenticate it, and treat pain before it gets worse.

Pain management has only recently become a recognized field of study. It is now accepted in the medical profession that pain resembles a disease of its own and that left alone, ignored, and untreated, pain will become more intense. Our bodies have a "pain memory" at a cellular level. A 1997 study at the University of Toronto compared the pain responses of groups of infant boys who had been circumcised with and without anesthetic. Four to six months later, the group without anesthetic had a lowered pain threshold, crying more at their first vaccination than those who had been anesthetized during circumcision. This and similar studies have led to the conclusion that there is a cellular memory of pain.

With a remembered pain sensation and with new pain, the effect on a patient can be traumatizing. It can worsen unless you are able to locate an empathetic, knowledgeable physician with a competent team of pain-management specialists to help.

Control Pain Early

Pain will often arrive without warning. Because we are socialized to fight pain and conquer it, it may take weeks or even months of our attempts to ignore it before we realize that pain has secured a permanent place in our lives. By this time, it has created a monster—a tired, angry, fretful, and passive victim. It is best to realize that pain needs attention early. To manage pain:

- Recognize and acknowledge it when your pain begins.
- Seek help early from your physician or pain-management specialist.
- Be active in the management process.
- Avoid allowing your tolerance level to increase.

Ask your doctor about pain clinics and treatment centers, and inquire whether or not she is willing to help you manage your pain. If you have difficulty locating a suitable pain center nearby, check the web sites on pages 167–68 for suggestions of somewhere close. In many cases, the pain center in your state can analyze your needs and give you a prescription that you can implement closer to home.

Pain is no longer managed simply with drugs. Water exercises, acupuncture, massage, physical therapy, biofeedback, electrical stimulation, and light exercise, such as that of tai chi or qi gong, serve as a backstop for a targeted, managed pain-control regimen.

And remember, be active in your care. Pain does make us passive. It requires extra effort from us to become active in its management. If your physician is planning to handle your pain only with medication, inquire about alternative treatments. Find out about the best licensed alternative or complementary medicine clinics in your city. Ask about massage, acupuncture, visualization, biofeedback training, and other healthful ways to relieve the pain in your body. And, if your doctor feels it is appropriate, work with him or her to find the least amount of medication that will work in partnership with your own body care. Read everything you can find about Eastern and Western medicine for pain. At the end of this chapter you will find recommended reading that specializes in pain education.

The pain of SjS is exhausting. We believe there are strategies to subdue it.

Fatigue

Fatigue, complete exhaustion, for an extended period of time, may be the first sign that you have SjS. It is not the fatigue that comes after doing something strenuous; rather this is a lack of energy even when doing the easiest most commonplace tasks. Particularly if fatigue lasts for three to four months and represents a dramatic change, it should alert you and

> Lately I feel dog tired all the time. I'm stressed with worry and feel very much alone. I think my family blames me. They think I'm just lazy, so there's no one to help and support me. Because I am always tired, I have had to take time off, and I am not making as much money as I did and I worry what will happen if I can't work at all. This worry and the fatigue have taken my life away. I'm sure it will get worse. All of this has colored my thinking about my future.
>
> —Amy

your physician to the need for referral to a rheumatologist. By fatigue, we do not mean tiredness, muscle weakness, pain, or stiffness. We speak of fatigue that includes all or some of these as well as a lack of interest in daily activities, a "brain fog" and an *overwhelming desire* to simply crawl onto a flat surface, curl up, and go to sleep—which happens repeatedly throughout the day and night. This is not a part of life; fatigue like this should be assessed and is not "just depression."

FATIGUE IS NOT JUST BEING TIRED

Fatigue affects everyone in a different way. Perhaps it is like this:

- Inertia. No energy. All you want is to sleep.
- Intense pain. Lowered pain threshold.
- Inability to concentrate. What some call "brain fog."
- Inability to plan, perform daily activities. A desire to just sleep.
- Irritability. Inability to be patient with loved ones and coworkers.

Many people, when confronted with extreme fatigue and looking for a diagnosis, may believe they suffer from chronic fatigue syndrome or fibromyalgia. CFS, like fibromyalgia, has been a catchall for unexplained fatigue, but there are some guideposts that can be used to assess the likelihood of its presence.

CHRONIC FATIGUE SYNDROME (CFS)

The symptoms of CFS include severe, unexplained fatigue that is not relieved by rest and has an identifiable onset (i.e., not lifelong fatigue). It must be persistent or relapsing fatigue that lasts for at least six or more consecutive months. It also must include four or more of the following symptoms:

- impaired memory or concentration problems
- tender cervical or axillary lymph nodes in neck
- sore throat (but may not show signs of infection)
- muscle pain
- multijoint pain (but not arthritis)
- new onset headaches (tension type or migraine)
- unrefreshing sleep (wake up in the morning feeling unrested)
- postexertional malaise (fatigue, pain, and flulike symptoms after exercise)

Fibromyalgia

Fibromyalgia is a syndrome of diffuse pain often present for years and often accompanied by subjective complaints such as fatigue, memory difficulties, sleep disturbance, and irritable bowel symptoms. It is characterized by trigger/tender points (mentioned in Chapter 8) and normal laboratory studies. Fibromyalgia is an accepted diagnosis when there is widespread pain which has been present for three months, pain in all four quadrants of the body, pain in one of eighteen specific tender points, and discomfort when eight pounds of pressure are applied to one of those tender points. The indeterminate nature of the symptoms and the fact that all of them may not be present at one time make diagnosis difficult. SjS can be present; if so, it manifests as dry eyes and dry mouth. If present with fibromyalgia, it would be considered primary Sjögren's syndome since fibromyalgia is not recognized as an autoimmune disorder. The diagnosis should be applied only after a thorough exclusion of other possible diagnoses. Too often the label is given to patients with chronic pain without proceeding with a thorough investigation for other explanations. The cause of fibromyalgia is not known. SjS can be distinguished from CFS because SjS does not cause recurrent sore throats (pharyngitis) and from fibromyalgia because SjS often will have autoantibodies or a characteristic minor salivary gland biopsy, both of which are not present in fibromyalgia.

The fatigue related to active immune disease is now generally attributed to central nervous system action of cytokines such as IL-1 or TNF, which were mentioned in Chapter 1. Tests such as the C-reactive protein test and sedimentation rate test are a good measure of their activity.

The first step in diagnosis is to rule out certain other possible causes: that the fatigue is not related to a hormonal imbalance or inflammation or caused by nonimmune, nonhormonal problems. Fatigue is also associated with hypothyroidism and anemia, both of which can be detected with a simple blood test.

Fatigue that comes with lack of sleep, for whatever reason—depression, anxiety, waking in the night because of thirst or a need to urinate—can plague you throughout the day. If the sleeplessness originates with the inflammation of SjS, certain medications to tame the systemic manifestations of the disorder could help calm your system and ultimately bring back the pleasure of a good night's rest.

TREATMENT OF FATIGUE

Both emotional and physical rest are essential to enjoyment of everyday life for someone with SjS. If the cause is inflammation, your physician may suggest hydroxycholorquine (Plaquenil) or possibly low-dose glucocorticoid (prednisone), each of which could have side effects but may reduce inflammation and enable you to return to a more balanced state and perhaps even improve your quality of sleep. Occasionally, in severe SjS cases, more potent immunomodulators such as azathioprine (Imuran) may be used.

The increased need for rest is not imaginary. So often we and members of our family and coworkers belittle the need for sleep. You are well advised, however, to be good to yourself and respect your need for rest and sleep. You will feel better with rest periods spaced throughout the day and longish sleeps at night. Restful sleep for eight to ten hours each night is a basic need for everyone and even more so for those with autoimmunity. A recent study of sleep needs at Pennsylvania State College of Medicine by Alexandros N. Vgontzas, M.D., et al. indicates that sleeping only six hours each night is associated with a change of blood factors that activates the inflammation process as well as increases daytime sleepiness and decreases performance.

Emotional rest is needed too. Emotional stressors can trigger a "flare" of SjS. Simple everyday things—noise, other people's demands, driving in traffic—cause stress; finding ways to avoid or reduce the stressors in life is essential. And remember that another person's definition of stress may be quite different from yours. It sounds platitudinous to repeat emotional dictums, but if you try reining in the stress in your life, even just for a short while, you may be surprised to discover that the physical signs of your illness improve. A quiet darkish place that you can use as a retreat is the first requirement. Then, make it clear to everyone that this is your needed "downtime." And make sure you practice self-care by setting aside a peaceful time in your day every day. Even closing the door while you lunch is a start. A walk in the park is refreshing, and fifteen minutes of your favorite music is a perfect way to center yourself away from the demands of others; even pleasant demands can still provide stress. Stress may also be the result of negative thought patterns, so taking time to reflect can catch those attacks of negative thoughts.

You might consider asking for a referral to an occupational therapist who can come to your home and workplace to help set up an "energy-conserving environment."

There are courses in meditation and disease offered by most hospitals. Review your library shelves for books on stress reduction. An excellent place to begin is Jon Kabat-Zinn's book *Wherever You Go, There You Are: Mindfulness Meditation in Everyday Life.* In Chapter 9 of this book, "The Emotional Toll of Chronic Disease," we will explore these issues in further detail.

Try some planning strategies to help manage your fatigue:

- Use your fatigue as an early warning system and be extra careful with your activities on those days when fatigue is at its worst.
- Plan ahead. Prepare a task list (even in your head) and follow it carefully.
- Make sure you have set aside two or three "downtimes" throughout the day.
- Combine tasks so that you don't double up on trips.
- Sit when working and use tools that take less energy.
- Tell your friends when you may or may not be able to visit with them. Be honest! They need to hear from you if they are going to be helpful.
- Follow a gentle exercise program, making sure that you do this throughout the day and not just before bed. Morning is best.
- Get enough sleep. If you are restless, ask your doctor for suggestions. Perhaps a medication can be used for a short time to get you in the sleep groove again.

And finally, if you notice that symptoms of pain and fatigue plague you after a viral or bacterial infection, it could be that this is simply the process by which your body adjusts. Often this "flare" will abate about six weeks after the worst of the infection has passed. Practice your coping strategies and keep track of the time. You may just take a while longer than you would like to recover.

Both pain and fatigue are a part of SjS. What we would like to advocate here is the idea that they need attention, respect, and management and that well-being can follow.

Recommended Reading

The Chronic Pain Solution: Your Personal Path to Pain Relief: The Comprehensive, Step by Step Guide to Choosing the Best of Alternative and Conventional Medicine (New York: Bantam, 2002), by James N. Dillard, M.D., D.C., C.Ac., is an excellent guide by a practitioner of Western and alternative medicine. Easy to read and understand, it helps a patient choose from among the best sources of alternative and conventional medicine.

Mayo Clinic on Chronic Pain, published by the Mayo Clinic (1999), is well written and easy to read.

Arthritis Foundation's Guide to Alternative Therapies, written by Judith Horstman and published by the Arthritis Foundation (1999), is a comprehensive resource for the healing systems, diet and exercise, and mind/body treatments that are available to treat chronic pain. It offers an excellent overview for patients who want to understand all of the available options for healing. Available at *www.arthritis.org.*

The Relaxation and Stress Reduction Workbook (Atlanta: New Harbinger Press, 1998) by Martha Davis, Elizabeth Robbins Eshelman, and Matthew McKay offers techniques for reducing stress, managing pain, and coping with chronic illness.

CHAPTER 8

Special Considerations

Intimacy and Sjögren's Syndrome

Sexual difficulties are not easy to talk about in spite of the fact that pain during lovemaking is common to sufferers of Sjögren's syndrome. It is embarrassing, and even though it would be helpful to share similar experiences, dryness that causes painful intercourse is rarely discussed. Whether in a support group or between friends, the experience of discomfort during lovemaking is just too embarrassing to share. Nevertheless, patients with Sjögren's syndrome do experience difficulties with intercourse, external pain, vaginal dryness, and candida, or yeast infection. Many of these symptoms develop normally as women age but are exacerbated with SjS.

The cause of this deficit of moisture is a localized inflammatory process within the glandular tissue that leads to a decrease in quantity and quality of secretions. There is a lessening of the lubricating fluid to the vaginal wall. Knowing what causes it doesn't help make it better. Nor does worrying about it or becoming anxious. There is a lot you can do about sexual difficulties with SjS, the first of which is to become active in seeking care for yourself.

Whether you are just beginning a relationship, have a long-standing love affair with your mate, or simply feel the discomfort of dry tissue, your discomfort can be improved. Understand that vaginal dryness is very common. Even if you are menopausal or perimenopausal, you need not accept that this is a natural progression, that you are not entitled to an active, healthy sex life, or that this is the way things will remain.

With your resolve to find help, it is possible to find an understanding gynecologist who is conversant with the vagaries of autoimmunity. Your rheumatologist or primary-care physician could be your guide. Ask if she knows a physician who has helped other autoimmune patients of hers and make an appointment for an initial consultation. Check out your impressions. How you relate to one another is important. Does the physician make you feel comfortable? Since a gynecologist has heard it all before and wants to help, she should be empathetic and interested. If she is not, find someone else. Your gynecologist will assess your circumstances and rule out any physical problems that may be beyond your purview.

With the understanding you gain through this visit, your next step is a quiet thoughtful talk with your partner. The two of you can do a lot to improve lovemaking. If your reaction to this statement causes you to skip to the next section, try to think this through. There are many ways to be comfortable with talk about intimacy, not the least of which is your eagerness to return to the intimacy you experienced before the dryness intruded itself. If you can work together, so much the better, but if not, there are many personal strategies your gynecologist can suggest.

Ask yourself whether or not the tissue feels elastic and moist. If not, there are creams and gels to make daily life and intercourse more enjoyable. There are moisturizing gels to be used for personal comfort. There are greaseless and colorless lubricating gels that can be used for arousal and intercourse. There are medicated creams for specific problems that are only available from your doctor. Discuss vaginal moisturizers, perhaps products like Feminease by Parnell, which contains yerba santa, or Silken Secret by Astroglide, made by Biofilm Inc., and K-Y Silk.

You may also wonder about hormone-replacement therapy (HRT). The disease process of Sjögren's patients causes atrophic vaginitis, so vaginal dryness and infectious overgrowth are potentially more of a problem. Since this is more a quality-of-life issue than a potential life-threat, physicians may tend to be inattentive when you raise it. It is wise to persist. There are medical treatments that can improve your symptoms and overall health. For some patients, a topical estrogen cream could be recommended. For others there are local dispensers of low-dose estradiol, such as the patch or ring, that can improve the symptoms. The Women's Health Initiative findings caused a disruption in the understanding of hormone-replacement therapy. Since this is an individual matter for the patient and since there are alternative methods of delivery and dosages, this is a subject that should be discussed thoroughly with your specialist. When autoimmunity is present, every drug intervention must be monitored by your physician, so make certain that you are monitored when on HRT. Physicians now need to discuss the pros and cons of HRT extensively with each and every patient. Balancing all the benefits and risks needs to be an individual decision based on your own research and the informed advice of your doctor.

Candida, a yeast overgrowth that can appropriate drying tissue, can be troubling. While advertisements seem to say that a cure is as simple as one, two, three, that is not the case. Your physician will take a culture sample of your tissue and prescribe the appropriate treatment—but only, we say again, if you bring it up.

None of these are life-threatening problems, but they can seriously mar the joy in your relationship. Talking with your partner and with a gynecologist will restore your sensuality and allow you to have the intimacy that you need and desire.

Pregnancy and Sjögren's Syndrome

What is simply "the dryness disease" may become more serious when you plan to have a family. It is well recognized that a small percentage of babies born to mothers with SSA and SSB antibodies are at risk for congenital heart block. It is also known that the same mother can have normal babies while giving birth to siblings who suffer in this way. While the phenomenon has been noted, the process of its occasion is unknown. Congenital heart block in a newborn can be related to SSA (Ro) antibodies, which cross from the mother through the placenta to the child and are associated with this serious conduction abnormality. Antibodies can also be associated with myocarditis in the newborn.

No book, and certainly not this one, can advise you on this most serious matter. The personal care that you need is beyond the scope of a book like this. Luckily there are specialists who can monitor your progress and advise you on each step during pregnancy. We do know that antibodies, which normally protect against invasion by foreign bodies such as viruses and bacteria, cross the placenta at about the end of the first trimester of pregnancy. Since there is no mechanism for the fetus to stop the SjS antibodies, they are transported through the placenta and enter the circulatory system of the infant. The resulting illness is deceptively known as *neonatal lupus*. The derivation of the term relates to infants born to autoimmune-affected women who develop a facial rash characteristic of the facial coloration of adults with systemic lupus erythematosus (SLE). Because many mothers do not have symptoms but carry the SSA/SSB antibodies and/or additional autoantibodies, the first indication of difficulty could be the diagnosis of an autoimmune disorder in the newborn baby. These transported antibodies can be harmful to the fetus or newborn infant. They can affect the heart, blood, skin, and liver, and, the most serious and most common of all, they can cause a complete congenital heart block. Because everything that happens while you are carrying a child needs monitoring, it is imperative that you seek experienced counsel early, preferably before you become pregnant. We can tell you what happens in general, but you will need to consult your physician every step of the way. Plan ahead: seek an obstetrician who is specified as perinatologist or "high-risk physician."

Such a physician can advise you as to the best time to become pregnant. She and her team will monitor you during pregnancy. It is important to let your caretakers know if you or your family has a history of autoimmunity and if abnormal antibodies have been found previously. Since heart block, if it develops, will not show up in the ordinary testing/ultrasound, when you come in for a checkup, the physician will check whether the fetal heart beat is below normal for a fixed amount of time and from that judge whether there is a heart block. The team will regularly monitor the fetal heart rate to ascertain whether or not the baby is developing normally. As you come closer to the thirty-second week, the monitoring will be increased to twice a week. Some physicians suggest that these tests begin earlier. They look for a healthy placenta, sufficient amniotic fluid, and a good weight gain for the baby. The baby's lungs are checked along with other vital signs. At the thirty-sixth week, the doctor begins to think of early delivery—always by cesarian section. Heart block, if it is to occur, usually does so at the thirty-sixth or thirty-seventh week of pregnancy. Since the placenta changes at about this time and since we know that once the baby is free of the placenta, he or she will be free of risk, it is reasonable to have an early delivery. Whatever antibodies have made it to the infant will dissipate over a few weeks. So with patience and support the problem resolves, and the baby can develop normally with most of the autoantibodies, except those associated with the heart block.

The prognosis for these babies, once they have been stabilized with good pediatric care, is mostly good. The heart block, if it develops, is permanent and is treated with a pacemaker that can be implanted in infancy. There is no indication that the child will develop SjS or SLE. As we said earlier, the process for the development of congenital heart block is still a mystery, but research is ongoing and hopefully will yield helpful results soon. The Hospital for Joint Diseases–Orthopedic Institute in New York City is actively pursuing studies into the causes and eventual eradication of this problem. The physicians there are enlisting patients who are at risk and whose children have been affected to participate in whatever way they can. The National Research Registry of Neonatal Lupus is a clearinghouse of affected patients and the center of interest for this condition. Information on the proportion of children requiring pacemakers, mortality, and recurrence rates in a subsequent pregnancy is critical for family counseling, research strategies, and management. The National Research Registry for Neonatal Lupus was initiated in September 1994 to establish a database of mothers whose children have complete congenital heart block (CHB) and/or other manifestations (dermatologic, hepatic, hematologic) of neonatal lupus. They welcome physician referrals of eligible patients.

If you are interested in further discussion of the problems of pregnancy with positive SjS antibodies, you might try the Sjögren's Syndrome Foundation chat list—SS-L—found at the foundation's web site. Once you sign up, look in the archives for "pregnancy." See page 168 for the URL.

Men and Children Have Sjögren's Syndrome Too!

While the number of male sufferers of SjS is small—just 9 to 10 percent of diagnosed cases—the intensity of the disorder in men is just as great as that in women. The symptoms seem to be different, however. Men do not seem to have the nonexocrine glandular disturbances, the main complaints being

Jeremy was seven on the day he called me from a soccer game to come and pick him up because he felt really sick. And when I did, I noticed that one side of his face was swollen; it looked as if he had mumps. But hadn't he been immunized against mumps when he was a baby? The doctors assured me that the vaccination doesn't always work and that it would be best if he had it again. Along with the immunization, they gave him high-dose antibiotics for the swelling. It slowly went down, and he began to feel better. We relaxed, although I had misgivings.

Unfortunately, my misgivings were well founded. A few months later, he had a repeat of the swelling and illness. Again the ear, nose, and throat specialist gave him antibiotics, explaining that it looked like parotiditis. Perhaps, he thought, it was caused by an allergy. This experience repeated itself as Jeremy turned eight and then nine years old.

After the fourth flare-up, when the antibiotics made him so ill that he was off school for two weeks, I asked for more tests. I was refused. Not satisfied, I took him to the hospital nearby and, luckily, found a doctor there who tested him for every possibility. It was then that his blood work came back with indicators of autoimmunity and a diagnosis of SjS.

You have no idea what having a diagnosis did to our family. I realize that SjS is uncommon in children but it does happen. I fault those doctors who didn't follow the signs and test him properly. He had so many months of unnecessary suffering, and we had so many months of anxiety.

Now Jeremy is under the care of an excellent rheumatologist, and he has had fewer problems since then. Having an understanding ear when something unexpected crops up has helped enormously.

—Sylvia

a lack of moisture in the eyes and mouth. However, men may not seek help as often as women do, so we do not have an accurate assessment of the spectrum of the disease in men and boys. Men are less likely to visit physicians for disease management and may suffer more than women because of this.

SjS, although rare, is known to manifest in children. Its rarity limits the information we are able to gather about its incidence, diagnosis, or treatment. It often appears as fatigue and swollen glands. It is often misdiagnosed as mumps.

Sadly, Jeremy's story above is not unique. Children with autoimmune conditions are rarely diagnosed early in their illness. Pediatric rheumatologists are skilled in the evaluation of childhood chronic rheumatic diseases;

the problem is recognizing that such a referral is needed. Check with the American Medical Association for a pediatric rheumatologist in your city or state. Go to the web site for the American Medical Association, click on "doctor finder" and expand their list of specialties. Pediatric rheumatology is in the expanded list of specialties. If your city does not have a doctor with this specialty, expand the search to your state, or consider finding an adult rheumatologist who is familiar with treating children through the American College of Rheumatology web site: *www.rheumatology.org*— "find a rheumatologist."

Of special consideration in childhood cases of SjS is meticulous dental care: frequent rinsing and brushing, and regular dental visits, as well as avoiding high-sugar and sticky snacks. Dental sealants can reduce the chance of early decay. Children may not complain about eye dryness until they experience pain, so regular screening, use of eye drops, and sunglasses should be recommended. Many children and adolescents do not like to feel "different" by having to observe these preventive measures, so a clear discussion about the reasons as well as an explanation of the consequences are essential. A reward for compliance can go a long way. Schools should be an ally in carrying out the program, for example, by allowing the child to keep a water bottle on the desk and by administering eye drops at recess (there are several laws mandating this kind of assistance).

Allergy and Sjögren's Syndrome

Although the link between allergy and autoimmunity has not been studied intensively, anecdotal evidence seems to suggest that an increased number of upper-respiratory infections occur when an underlying allergy exists. In SjS, the mucous-membrane-protective barrier is defective. It is dry. Allergic reactions can exacerbate things. These forces—dry, receptive tissue and allergic inflammation—could explain this increase in infectious processes that occurs in some SjS patients. And allergy symptoms are usually controlled with antihistamine medications, which are drying themselves, thereby creating a nonstop cycle of dryness and disease.

Recently, Singulair, an asthma medication that was prescribed over the flu season as preventive, has been found to prevent the frequency of these infections, lessening the need for repeated antibiotic medications.

Secondary Sjögren's Syndrome

There is no accurate count of the number of patients with secondary SjS. An accepted estimate suggests that one half of those diagnosed with SjS can be said to have secondary Sjögren's syndrome. That means that half of the 4 million cases in the United States with SjS suffer with it along with another autoimmune disorder. The most common of these are rheumatoid arthritis, scleroderma, and lupus (SLE).

Rheumatoid arthritis, primarily a disease of the joints, can affect other organ systems in the body. While RA is characterized by joint pain and swelling and possibly boney destruction (erosions), one should remember that anemia, fever, and fatigue can also be present. Problems can arise in other organs, such as the heart, lungs, skin, and eyes. When the lacrimal and salivary glands become inflamed, that patient is said to suffer from rheumatoid arthritis with secondary SjS.

Systemic lupus erythematosus, known as lupus, is a chronic disease that can affect the entire body. Those who endure the pain, fatigue, and unpredictability of lupus also suffer a roller coaster of feelings and disability. When dry eyes and mouth are present, SjS probably has entered the picture. A comprehensive rheumatologic diagnostic evaluation will help establish this possibility. The Lupus Foundation, Sjögren's Syndrome Foundation, and Arthritis Foundation all have excellent educational information to help you understand the workings of SLE and other disorders.

Scleroderma is a chronic autoimmune disease that can affect both the external (the skin) and internal organs. It is a tightening (fibrosing) of the skin due to an excess of collagen, the reason for which is unknown. When the internal organs are affected, the condition is extremely serious. It can affect almost any part of the body: heart, lungs, joints, gastrointestinal tract, muscles, and blood vessels. Early symptoms are similar to those of other autoimmune disorders: pain and stiffness in your joints, swelling of your hands and feet, GI troubles, fatigue, weakness, and aching. Since these symptoms sound so like those of other autoimmune disorders, it is important to have them checked by a rheumatologist. Scleroroderma can be complicated by SjS when eyes and mouth become dry—another case of secondary Sjögren's syndrome.

Autoimmune disorders are elusive and difficult to treat. Often, however, when you effectively treat the primary process, the symptoms of SjS are relieved.

Thinking of Disability?

Perhaps you need to apply to the Social Security Administration for disability and are unsure of how to begin. Or you have already applied and been turned down. Thanks to several chronic disease associations, we were referred to Physicians' Disability Services, Inc., and the *Disability Workbook for Social Security Applicants*.

It consolidates the information you need to fulfill your role in proving disability. It also includes steps you take to win an appeal to SSA if you have been turned down initially. The workbook is written by a disability lawyer and is updated regularly.

Check their web site for more information *www.disabilityfacts.com* or write to PDS, P.O. Box 827, Arnold, MD 21012, (410) 431-5279.

Recommended Reading

The New Sjogren's Syndrome Handbook, edited by S. Carsons, M.D., and Elaine Harris (New York: Oxford University Press, 1998). New edition soon.

Fibromyalgia & Chronic Myofascial Pain Syndrome, by Devin Starlanyl and Mary Ellen Copeland (Berkeley, Calif.: New Harbinger Press Inc., 1996).

The Emotional Toll of Chronic Disease

THOSE WHO SUFFER WITH CHRONIC ILLNESS FRE-
quently develop distressing emotional and psychological symptoms. The
feelings may wax and wane, even disappear at times, but for many an underlying sense of grief and loss may persist.

A book is not the appropriate venue for advising sufferers on how to
cope with such feelings; those seeking help should consult a therapist or
counselor. However, we believe it is essential to warn SjS patients of the
dangers of not recognizing and dealing with the feelings of sorrow and
anger that arise unbidden in response to chronic illness. Studies have
shown that hopefulness and optimism often may be as important to a patient's health as medications. Patients with a negative attitude will have
poorer health than those who look hopefully toward a future where symptoms will be manageable. It is particularly difficult to remain hopeful when
unexplained symptoms crop up or when pain and fatigue succeed in bury-
ing our good nature. The first step toward optimism and healing is to acknowledge our losses. Acknowledgment is a process, so perhaps the first
thing we need to do is recognize that this will take time and that it may be
difficult but that it is necessary. How much simpler just to stay in denial!

Mourning Our Losses

Denying the presence of an illness, or any troubling life issue for that matter, can be an effective coping mechanism for a while, but not coming to terms with it can ultimately have a detrimental effect on physical as well as emotional healing. It is important to get on with life, but stuffing the sadness inside will eventually backfire. Feelings of sorrow, loss, and anger will erupt, with results that may be even more devastating than the feelings themselves. Grieving for the person you once were is to be expected. After all, the person you once were has changed significantly, and you may long for her return. The natural response to the loss of good health is to mourn it as you would the loss of a friend. Mourning the loss of your good health is similar to mourning a death, except it is far lonelier. When someone you love dies, the mourning process is shared with your siblings, friends, and community. When you mourn the loss of your healthy self, you do it alone. You are the one who remembers what it felt like to have boundless energy, and you are the one who feels the lack of it. Mourning that loss is essential. If you are to reach an understanding and acceptance of this new life, you must first mourn the loss of the old.

Mourning the losses involved in a chronic disease process is an ongoing process in itself. Your physical abilities change as the disease changes. Unlike the death of a loved one, chronic illness brings about "mini deaths." These multiple and often underrecognized deaths may involve the loss of what you were once able to do physically, the loss of ways in which you defined yourself and gained your self-esteem, and the loss of hope for the future you had planned.

In 1969, Dr. Elisabeth Kübler-Ross wrote *On Death and Dying,* in which she hypothesized that grief is a five-stage process:

- denial to avoid grief
- anger to displace feelings
- bargaining to control grief
- depression to bury grief
- acceptance when we face grief and the future

While we don't follow each step in sequence, Dr. Kübler-Ross claimed that we weave in and out of each one, holding on to one as we experience another. With acceptance, the ultimate stage, we find comfort. Acceptance, does not mean necessarily that we welcome the disorder or that we ignore it. It means acknowledging the impact of the disorder on our lives while allowing ourselves, as much as possible, to continue on with the activities and tasks that contribute to the fullness of living. This may mean adopting certain activities or finding new ones that are better suited to our physical status. Acceptance is not a state of mind that magically happens as one deals with the effects of having a chronic disorder. We don't have to like what is happening to our bodies, but acceptance means being able to push the problems aside for long enough to move on with our lives. For many people, this challenge is presented on a daily basis and can require almost constant vigilance to prevent the symptoms from taking total control of their life. Acceptance means learning to live with our disorder in spite of resenting and hating its effects. At least, that is the hope for a healthy approach to our disorder. Let's see how these stages look when applied to SjS.

DENIAL

You say to yourself, "It was a mistake; I don't have this disorder. At least, I have a mild case, and it will go away." Or you tell yourself, "This doctor made a mistake. A few medications and I'll be fine—forever." Or you feel well for a while and exult, "I'm cured." But then, you're defeated; it returns.

ANGER

Anger is the natural result of this defeat—anger at everyone who is healthy, at yourself for being ill, at the disorder for its mystery, and at the family whose disappointment can't help but make it all worse. Anger, in this case, is a good thing. It is a great cathartic. Let her rip. Express your anger in any way that's best but be careful not to hurt yourself or others in the process. Explain to friends that you need to talk about how you feel. Buy some watercolors and large sheets of drawing paper and paint your pain away. Write your feelings in a journal. Go to a glass-recycling center and toss glass bottles into the bins. Hammer nails into a thick wood board. Pound on a pillow or a punching bag. The list goes on. Allow your imagination to roam until you find an outlet that is practical and effective for you. Above all, acknowledge that you feel anger and understand that it is appropriate. Be careful that your angry reaction does not turn inward and become self-destructive. Many of us are taught that anger is an unacceptable reaction, more so if there is nothing we can do about the situation that has provoked it, when it just doesn't seem to make sense, and when there is no clear entity with whom to get angry other than the disorder. Watch for attempts to push anger away, such as overeating or abusing alcohol. As difficult as it may be, the better route is to try to find outlets—psychotherapy, support groups, supportive friends—where you can express your rage in safety while being careful not to hurt the feelings of others.

BARGAIN

In the grieving process you may notice anger diminish as you begin to bargain: "I'll take all my medication, and the disorder will disappear." "If I give up my regular jogging sessions, I'll get better." Bargaining works—for a short while.

DEPRESSION

When all else fails, depression awaits. Depression is a normal reaction to loss. Unfortunately, when physical ailments are so disabling, emotional ones are often neglected. Many people who suffer from depression because of chronic illness will not seek help when it's needed. Depression is a clinical condition that is treatable, most commonly with psychotherapy and/or medication. It's the wise physician who looks for the signs of emotional stress, anxiety, and depression, and attempts to help her patient.

After a while, and with treatment, depression will abate. Eventually our thoughts will bring us to acceptance, a place where we might not like the disorder one bit, but where we can function as well as possible in our daily lives.

These five stages of grief provide a template for understanding the difficult and frequently lonely process of coming to grips with chronic illness. While no one can share them with you, you do not need to go through the process alone. In many respects, this is a solitary journey, but in others it is a shared one that will enable you to accept the change in your life and to move on with grace and dignity. You will come to accept that doctor's appointments will be a regular part of life, as will medications, rest, stress reduction, and gentle exercise.

ACCEPTANCE

Acceptance brings with it a willingness to let others help. Once others understand that this is a chronic condition that will not go away, that there are things that they can do to help, their own sense of worth will grow too. Your relationships will change. Allowing others to be there for you in various capacities to supply emotional as well as practical support can only bring you closer.

A Word About the "Blues"

Winston Churchill, famous for his bleak depression, gave it a nickname. It became known by family and friends as "his little black dog." We might take a leaf from his book and characterize our feelings with a descriptive phrase—even "the blues" works for some. It takes some experience to recognize a depression as it arises, because depression comes very gradually and unbidden. Depression skulks into our psyches with little warning. It is insidious and persistent. Soon we are sleeping more than usual, hibernating throughout the week and weekends, and taking little interest in daily activities. Since depression is now a treatable illness with clear signs and symptoms, and not just simple feelings of sadness we might be better served to do as Churchill did; recognize it, name it, and treat it.

Anyone can be a casualty of depression. Life events effect even the most hardy. It seems that it will never end and that there is no way out. What's more, we haven't the energy to do anything about it. So, you need to take this on faith and seek help. Professional help can make a difference!

You may be diagnosed with depression, if at least five of the following symptoms have been present during the same two-week period and represent a change from previous functioning, and at least one of the symptoms is either depressed mood or loss of interest or pleasure.

- depressed mood most of the day, nearly every day
- markedly diminished interest or pleasure in all, or almost all, activities most of the day, nearly every day
- significant weight loss or weight gain when not dieting
- insomnia or too much sleep every day
- agitation or slowing down

- fatigue or loss of energy nearly every day
- feelings of guilt or worthlessness
- diminished ability to think or concentrate, or indecisiveness, nearly every day
- suicidal thoughts or recurrent thoughts of death

If, in reading this, you think "hah, that's me!"—if you feel that you can't cope, that your relationships are suffering, that your work is over-whelming—bring it up with your doctor with the expectation of a referral to a psychotherapist. Treatment of depression includes medications of ad-equate dose and duration to help ease the feelings of sorrow that have brought you there. Talk therapy, whether with a psychiatrist, psychothera-pist, social worker, or clergyperson, will support you as you discover strate-gies for dealing with the ups and downs of SjS. Patients seem to benefit especially from cognitive-behavioral therapy, a type of therapy that deals with the here and now (you may be comforted to know that not all thera-pies are dependent on exploring family issues when you were three years old), as well as group and couples therapy.

Anxiety

Each new symptom brings a new fear. There are times when your fears are specific and relate to a particular new symptom. There are other times when you feel generalized anxiety with no traceable cause. In either case, you could experience shortness of breath or dizziness, palpitations, feelings of pending doom, and nausea or abdominal distress.

Again, there are treatments for these feelings. They include medication, psychotherapy, relaxation techniques, and support groups. Your physician is trained to understand the symptoms and treatments and will refer you to the appropriate professional for help. SjS is predicament enough; why continue with the psychological disorders that can be eased?

Sjögren's Syndrome Can Change Your Relationships

Intimacy suffers in the presence of chronic disorder. One can think of chronic illness as the "corespondent" in a marriage; it comes between you and your spouse, taking your attention and separating you, if not bodily, at least emotionally from one another. Having SjS is a bit like having a demanding, exacting, unpredictable but needy two-year-old in your life who is forever nagging for your attention.

Your partner's anger and frustration may seem to be directed at you rather than at your disease, which ultimately will bring about relationship problems. Keep in mind that with SjS, as with other chronic and unpredictable disorders, there is a third party present in your relationship—the disease—that must be acknowledged and adequately discussed.

For your loved one, be he partner, child, parent, friend, or husband, the disorder that snatches all your attention is the target of his or her anger and frustration. In yet another way, chronic disease changes your life.

We mentioned the five stages of grief earlier, but it's appropriate to mention them again here. It is likely that your spouse or partner suffers through them in much the same way that you do. The loss is tangible, and your partner will feel the same denial, anger, bargaining, depression, and finally, if you both persevere in your openness, acceptance. The process can repeat itself as the disorder waxes and wanes until finally, a sort of peace will settle on you, and you will be able to share in the process of getting and keeping well.

There are many roads you can travel as you grapple with SjS. Keeping your feelings hidden is not one of them. When you awaken with new symptoms that worry you, your inclination may be to "protect" your loved ones by keeping silent. But how will that affect the inflammatory process that is going on in your body? Not well. Depression and anxiety flourish in an environment of silence and isolation. Eventually that strategy erodes, and a simple statement of fact will relieve you and clear the air of uncertainty.

It certainly is not helpful to be overly anxious and emotional either. To relieve your fear and anxiety, try stating the facts. "I am feeling a new symptom right now, and I am worried and I hurt" is a simple statement of fact. If you have prepared your spouse with the supportive answers you need to get through a flare-up, he could respond with "I know, and I am so sorry you feel like this." Feeling his physical presence through this flare-up will confirm his emotional support and create a deeper sense of closeness, rather than distance and isolation. And with that support, you will become clearer about what you need to do to help deal with this new development and keep your worry in perspective—learn to control the worry so it doesn't control you. Perhaps it will be an antidepressant or a new medication or a day under the covers with a good book. Whichever you choose, having talked through your needs and expectations with your partner or other loved ones and having had them talk through theirs with you, you'll find that your healing will progress more quickly than before.

Perhaps it is time to join a support group. The *Moisture Seekers,* the newsletter of the Sjögren's Syndrome Foundation, lists the support groups in your area. If there isn't one nearby and you have the energy, perhaps talk with the Foundation about beginning one of your own. From personal experience, we have learned that each group takes time to evolve into the form that works best for its members. Give yourself time to adjust to the others and to the feelings they bring up. The East Bay Group took two years to settle into a pattern that worked well. Monthly meetings were not possible, probably because of the distances involved, and now we have fewer meetings, which are held in the home of a member, where each member talks about "what worked" for them in the past months. This positive attitude continues into the tea hour as members talk amongst themselves about issues that have been discussed earlier. According to Irene Mc., our group is more helpful to her than all of her treks to the doctor. And since so many men accompany their wives to these meetings, it was decided that they adjourn during our time together and have coffee and talk about spousal reactions to SjS.

If an SjS group is not possible for you, contact the patients' liaison at your local hospital. There are support groups, and one or the other of them might suit you. You might find others will benefit from hearing about SjS, and you will learn about different conditions that present health challenges to others.

If a group is not an option for you, join a chat group on-line. There are two SjS chats, one for feelings and connections and one for medical and treatment discussions. Both are treasure troves of friendships and information.

In all cases, whether for yourself, a partner, or other significant people in your life, psychological insights make a great difference in the way you relate to SjS.

Where Do I Look for Help?

There are professionals trained and experienced in several disciplines who support the emotional needs of patients. Psychiatrists are medical doctors with additional training in psychological disorders. They are board certified and can be located through your physician and health plan. They can prescribe antidepressant and anxiety medications. Clinical psychologists have earned a doctorate in psychology and can be identified by the letters Ph.D. (Doctor of Philosophy) or Psy.D. (Doctor of Psychology) following their name. In addition there are many very competent therapists who have either M.A. (Master of Arts in psychology), M.S. (Master of Science), M.S.W. (Master of Social Work), or M.F.T. (Master of Family Therapy) following their names and degrees. Each person within a specialty—social work, psychology, psychiatry, or family therapy—is required to have a valid license from the appropriate state licensing board. Only psychiatrists, physicians who have been trained to understand the physical as well as emotional workings of our bodies and psyches, can prescribe medications.

Some insurers cover the whole or partial cost of treatment. This means that your choice of therapist will be limited to those on their lists. It also means that the insurers decide, in concert with the therapist, on the number of therapeutic visits covered under your plan. You may need to begin your search for help with the insurance company, but be sure to double-check with friends and your doctor before making the final decision. Seek referrals from your rheumatologist, probe friends or coworkers, and when you are satisfied with your choice, make an appointment to see how you feel with this person before deciding to continue. Since you are dealing with a chronic illness, it would be wise to stipulate this up front. Many professionals, having had an illness themselves or having had experience helping others with an illness, will have a particular interest and expertise in helping you. Often, therapists will offer a reduced rate for a first visit in order for you (and she) to evaluate whether or not the two of you are a good "fit." We realize the realities of the marketplace in some parts of the country will not allow you the freedom to choose; however, this is the recommended and most reliable way to find the right therapist for you.

Whomever you choose, keep clear about your need to feel better and more hopeful. If your work together does not achieve this and you are still feeling blue or anxious after six to ten visits, perhaps you should think of looking for someone else. Therapists want you to get better, and if you discuss your feelings openly, they will help you find someone else or adjust their treatment to better meet your needs.

SOME COPING STRATEGIES

- Take one day at a time. Taking on the whole disorder can feel overwhelming to anyone. On difficult days, you may have to take one minute at a time.
- Remind yourself that *you are not your disorder.* It may be affecting you and your ability to function, but you are more than your symptoms.
- Get help. Sadness, depression, and anxiety will thrive in an environment of isolation and embarrassment. Seek help from a close friend, family member, clergyperson, or psychotherapist. Antidepressant and antianxiety medications can help take the edge off disturbing and immobilizing reactions and feelings. Consult a psychiatrist to determine what best suits your needs.
- Get involved in a support group. Hearing how others cope will give you a sense of support and community. At best, it may give you a regular place to go where others truly and personally understand your problems. At worst, you will meet some interesting people and make new friends.
- Take excellent care of yourself. Consult with your doctor to see if an adaptive exercise program is appropriate for you. There are many strengthening exercises that can be done in an armchair at a slow pace to help maintain physical tone and endurance while helping you feel better about yourself.
- Most important, don't play "dead." Try to remind yourself every morning when you waken that you are alive and functioning the best you can at the moment. It is a tough task, like a balancing act, trying not to minimize the effects of your disorder while encouraging yourself to move on with life, but it can be done.

CHAPTER 10

Medications for Sjögren's Syndrome

THE MAJORITY OF SJÖGREN'S SYNDROME PATIENTS who suffer with dry eyes and mouth find that topical treatment with drops, gels, and lotions, and a preventive dental strategy is all they need. But for those with symptoms of muscle pain, joint pain, fatigue, and malaise, medications become a powerful line of offense and, when used cautiously, can be the difference between feeling sick and being well. They can also offer a brief intervention strategy that may assist the body in getting back into balance.

Western society has become accustomed to treating illness with medications that make us well quickly. We are unaccustomed to having to balance medications with side effects and choose between pain and other difficulties, and we are impatient with anything beyond a "quick-fix" cure. With autoimmunity there is no quick fix. Rather, what works is a thoughtful collaboration between a caring physician and an informed patient who discuss and initiate a program of medications that minimizes side effects. Furthermore, this strategy reduces the likelihood of developing tolerance to the therapy. A medication that has worked may stop working or a stronger dose of the medication may be needed to maintain its beneficial effect. An on-off strategy may allow an effective therapy to be used for a longer period of time with fewer side effects. Lower doses may minimize side effects. The strategy needs to be tailored to the individual; there are no large clinical trials to guide us.

Medication Management

We recommend a booklet, available without charge from the Arthritis Foundation through their web site, that will help you to become an informed consumer. It is the *Arthritis Today 2002 Drug Guide,* a twenty-six-page listing of various drugs that are prescribed for arthritic disorders and fibromyalgia, with comments, special instructions, possible side effects, cautions, and considerations for each category and each medication. Consider, too, that the Internet is a bountiful resource for the latest information about drugs; we have listed several excellent drug information web sites on pages 170–71.

As you and your doctor begin a treatment plan, try to establish realistic goals for your health management. The physician is looking to improve your quality of life by reducing inflammation, suppressing immune-system abnormalities, preventing flare-ups, and minimizing possible complications. This may mean that in order to avoid uncomfortable side effects you won't be able to completely eliminate your pain or other disability.

It seems that those with SjS and other chronic illnesses have a lower tolerance for medications and may have stronger reactions to them than others do. Think about beginning a new medication when you are least likely to be called upon for business decisions or carpooling, so that you can be alert to whatever body and mood changes occur. For example, it would be prudent to avoid beginning a new medication before leaving on vacation. Also consider the time you take the medication. It can further minimize potential negative effects.

Some medications have fewer side effects if taken at night. Methotrexate, for example, which is usually taken once a week, can bring on a mild nausea or headache, so try taking the medication before bed. Another example is a medication used to prevent steroid-induced osteoporosis—bisphosphonates (Fosamax, Actonel)—which must be taken thirty minutes before any food or other medications and requires that you remain upright during this time to avoid ulceration of the esophagus. All of this may not be practical during the week, when you are getting the family ready to start the day or rushing off to work, but on a weekend morning that same thirty minutes could be a gift, a welcome quiet time to read the paper or practice meditation.

If you have questions about the timing of your medications, we suggest you review it with your doctor. The goal here is to minimize potential side effects and follow a routine that works for you. And keep the doctor informed about your medication reactions and changes. If you stop for any reason, your doctor should be informed.

Medications frequently used to control symptoms are over-the-counter topical aids; nonsteroidal anti-inflammatory drugs (NSAIDs), both over the counter and by prescription; systemic medications for dry mouth, such as Salagen and Evoxac, which were discussed in Chapter 6; glucocorticoids; antimalarials; and disease-modifying antirheumatic drugs (DMARDs). And there are some experimental drugs being tested that are not yet in current use but that hold promise.

Over-the-Counter Topical Medications

This group includes eye drops and gels, mouth and nose moisteners, and liquids to thin mucous secretions. They are mild and have few side effects other than the discomfort that comes when they are not used regularly. For more information on topical medications for the eyes, see Chapter 4; for medications for the mouth, see Chapter 5.

Nonsteroidal Anti-inflammatories (NSAIDs)

OVER THE COUNTER

NSAIDs include medications like aspirin, ibuprofen (Advil, Motrin IB, Nuprin), and naproxen sodium (Aleve). NSAIDs have the ability to inhibit the release of prostaglandins that are responsible for producing inflammation and pain. There are side effects with these medications, and they should not be taken for an extended period of time without constantly checking to see if they work as you expect and have no untoward effects. Laboratory tests every several months for liver and kidney function may be indicated while you take any of these medications on a regular basis. NSAIDs can cause gastric problems and should be taken with food, antacids, or milk. If you suffer from mild muscle or joint pain and swelling, you will benefit from these medications; when the problem becomes persistent and more intense, you may need something stronger.

PRESCRIPTION

Prescription nonsteroidal anti-inflammatories, including naproxen (Naprosyn), diclofenac sodium (Voltaren), and ibuprofen (Motrin), are anti-inflammatories that require a doctor's prescription and supervision before they are taken for an extended period. There are some fifteen or so NSAIDs, and they work in your body in slightly different ways, and some work better for some people than others. Your physician will help decide which to try and will monitor your condition for any systemic problems. Check in with your rheumatologist and review how you are feeling every three months or so. The adverse effects of NSAIDs can be painful and dangerous: dyspepsia, heartburn, stomach distress, and nausea, even GI bleeding.

Recently new drugs that interfere with the Cox-1 and Cox-2 (cyclo-oxygenase) enzymes of our bodies have appeared on the market. Older, traditional NSAIDs reduce pain and inflammation by blocking the Cox-2 enzyme. However, they also inhibit Cox-1, the enzyme that helps maintain the lining of the stomach. The action against Cox-1 results in unwanted side effects such as stomach irritation and ulcers. This new class of NSAIDs, the Cox-2 inhibitors, selectively inhibit Cox-2 and spare Cox-1, thereby relieving pain and inflammation with less potential for gastrointestinal side effects. Both celecoxib (Celebrex) and rofecoxib (Vioxx) belong to the Cox-2 drug class.

There is a newer drug called valdecoxib (Bextra) on the market. Bextra has recently been associated with severe allergic skin reactions, and since many SjS patients are prone to various skin problems, it makes sense to start with Vioxx or Celebrex. If you have a history of allergy to sulfa drugs, the use of Celebrex needs to be carefully reviewed by your physician. There are more drugs like this in development, but they are not yet on the market. If you are at risk for stroke or heart attack, you would be advised to continue to take low-dose aspirin every day. Cox-2 drugs don't have the same vascular advantage as the older NSAIDs; that is why they are easier on the GI tract and cause less bleeding. There has been some concern over increased risks of cardiovascular disease with the newer Cox-2 inhibitors, possibly because patients tended to stop the low-dose aspirin once they began taking the Cox-2. If cardiovascular health is an issue, work with your doctor to include 81 mg of aspirin daily when taking the newer medications. Mobic, another drug new to the United States but used in Europe for over five years, blocks both Cox-1 and Cox-2 but is Cox-2 selective, meaning that you get the benefits of less toxicity to the GI tract but still have some antiplatelet effect for your cardiovascular system.

Plaquenil/Hydroxychloroquine

Hydroxychloroquine is an antimalaria drug. Antimalarials were first used during World War II because quinine, the drug for malaria, was in short supply. Scientists discovered that this group of medications could be used successfully for joint pain. Subsequently, it was established that they work well with other inflammatory disorders. The drug in this category that is prescribed most often is hydroxychloroquine sulphate (Plaquenil).

Plaquenil is the first thing most members of SjS support groups discuss when they get together because it can relieve so many symptoms. For many people, it eases joint pain, fatigue, and dry eyes. While everyone has a different reaction to the medication, generally, two points emerge about the effectiveness of Plaquenil: (1) It can help halt the progression of SjS, and (2) it often takes several months to become effective.

Physicians will usually recommend a three- to six-month initial trial, during which time the dose may need to be increased to determine benefit and maximal response. In the future, using higher doses than those currently used may shorten the response time. Like all medications, there are side effects, worse for some people than for others. Each individual will have a particular reaction to the drug. Side effects cannot be predicted although nausea and gastric upset have been reported.

Plaquenil is extremely well tolerated in most people. It is easy to take, and only rarely are there side effects. If you miss a few doses you will not lose any of the benefit since it is stored in your tissues and some will remain in your system even after stopping.

A recommended starting dose of Plaquenil is one pill (200 mg) every other day for 1 week, then daily for one week, then two pills per day (for a total dose of 400 mg). Lower doses may be required for very sensitive people. A good strategy would be to finely grind the tablet and sprinkle it on cereal, gradually increasing the dose over time. Personal observation indicates that the brand-name form of the drug is more easily tolerated than the generic for some patients who are able to bear the former while rejecting the latter. This could possibly have something to do with the bioavailability of the generic form of the drug or the sensitivity of the patient to the filler compounds that are used to form it into a tablet.

Some people are allergic to Plaquenil and develop body rash and itching. If this is the case, report it to your doctor, who may recommend that you reduce the dose or add an allergy medication to your drug arsenal. Or discontinue the drug completely. It is wise to discontinue the drug if this happens until you review it with your physician. Individuals who have an enzyme deficiency called *G-6-P-D deficiency* are more prone to allergic reactions. Your physician can perform a test for this deficiency before starting the drug.

When taking Plaquenil, you will need clinical assessment of your eye condition. It is known that Plaquenil retinopathy causes loss in central vision, which results in color defects, decreased visual acuity, and central visual field defects. If you remain on Plaquenil for six to twelve months or longer it will be recommended that you see an ophthalmologist for a baseline exam and at least every year take tests for visual field and color along with a routine eye exam. Problems are rarely seen today with the current doses used. Your eye doctor can prevent problems by adjusting the dose or discontinuing the medication prior to the development of any clinical problem. If you develop new visual symptoms, such as flashing lights, you should stop the medication, let your prescribing physician know, and see your ophthalmologist shortly.

It is advisable to stay out of the sun when taking Plaquenil. If you are taking a tropical vacation, use sunscreen and sun-protective clothing; some physicians will suggest that you just stop the medication to avoid the increased sun sensitivity. Dosage is based on lean body weight, not real body weight. If you have fatty tissue, which raises your weight, the doctor will base your dosage, not on your scale weight but on your ideal weight as shown in the Insurance Tables of Weight and Height. It is dosed at 3 mg per pound of lean body weight. If you have adverse reactions to Plaquenil, check the dosage, and if it is correct (we assume it is), remind yourself that SjS patients have a lower tolerance for drugs. You may need to begin at a lowered dose with the expectation of increasing it. It is always advisable to take the lowest clinically effective dosage of any drug. Take Plaquenil before or after meals at the same time each day to maintain drug levels. If you are taking more than one pill, they may all be taken at the same time to make it easier to remember your pills.

Of all the drug options currently available, Plaquenil is the only one that has specific actions to down-regulate autoimmune hyperactivity with a minimal effect on normal immunity. It does not increase the risk of infections, such as colds and flu, as do steroids or immunosuppressive agents. Plaquenil decreases the level of inflammation and autoimmunity by:

- decreasing pro-inflammatory cytokines such as TNF-alpha and IL
- decreasing autoantigen presentation by the macrophage to the T-helper cell
- inhibiting the toll-like receptor-signaling pathway

Plaquenil has also been used to treat known viral infections such as hepatitis C and HIV without any untoward effects on the immune system or an increase in virally mediated disease. Since such patients may develop joint or other autoimmune problems, Plaquenil can provide some relief.

Glucosteroids

If there is one class of drug with which patients enjoy a love-hate relationship it is the group of glucocorticoids. There have been whole books written about the most commonly prescribed of these steroid medications: prednisone (Deltasone, Delta-Cortef, Prelone, Sterapred), hydrocortisone (Cortef, Hydrocortone), dexamethasone (Decadron, Hexadrol), and, intravenously administered, methylprednisolone (Solu-Medrol) and hydrocortisone (Solu-Cortef).

The "love" side of the relationship is related to the body's quick response to glucocorticoids. They efficiently relieve joint and muscle pain and fatigue, and suppress an overactive immune system by decreasing two broad arms of the immune system called the TH-1 and TH-2 response pathways. They ease inflammation of the joints and organs almost immediately and patients feel like they have returned to health.

Steroids are produced in the adrenal glands in the form of *cortisol*, a hormone that controls and affects numerous body functions. When additional steroid is added in the form of a medication, our adrenal glands decide to stop making cortisol. This happens over a period of time, and gradually the only cortisol available for normal functioning is the cortisol that comes in a pill. Once the adrenal glands have stopped putting out the hormone and the decision has been made to taper off the medication, the body finds itself in deficit. This can throw the body into a frenzy, with painful debilitating symptoms and even life-threatening problems with low blood pressure. When going off steroids, a patient must gradually taper back doses so the adrenals will slowly begin to produce cortisol again.

It is when steroid use is discontinued that the "hate" side of the relationship emerges. Reducing a steroid drug may bring back all the symptoms of the disorder plus the aching, weakness, and fatigue that is the result of the body's adjustment to varying levels of cortisol. To minimize these reactions, the dosage should be reduced gradually, and since no two people handle cortisol in the same way, test yourself and your reactions, but do it slowly. Some can reduce their dosage by 5 mg per week; some 5 mg every two weeks or even per month. Some patients need to make even smaller changes, 1 mg at a time.

The effect on the body when weaning off steroids can be strenuous. Often, when a dosage is reduced, patients feel that they will never return to their old self. But gradually, the body balances itself, and it can be reduced another milligram. The reaction is stronger at the lower doses because you are actually running on a cortisol deficit. This happens at doses around 7 mg per day. You need to persist as your adrenal gland boots up to produce more cortisol. The way in which some patients have made this easier is to go down 1 mg every other day. In other words, if you are at 5 mg on Monday, take 4 mg on Tuesday and 5 mg on Wednesday. Continue this protocol until you feel that your body is ready to remain on the lowered dose. Then repeat this with 3 mg, 2 mg, and finally 1 mg until you have completed the taper. Don't be surprised at how long it takes. It could be as long as one year before you have adjusted to having no additional glucocorticoid in your system. These dosage adjustments will of course be done in partnership with your rheumatologist, who will have additional recommendations to make it easier.

The decision to use these drugs is highly individualized and dependent upon the patient's condition. If there is organ involvement, if the patient is extremely ill, high-dose steroids will likely be prescribed. If it is a quality-of-life issue, both patient and doctor should seriously consider the side effects of the medication before a decision to prescribe is made. And when the medication is begun, glucosteroids should be taken with food every day at the same time.

Sometimes a short course of steroids will be considered to determine if the symptom complex unique to you is reversible with medication. The quickest way to get this answer is with a trial of steroids, using the dose that is effective as a guide to the choice of other agents. If a small dose (e.g., 5 mg/day) works, Plaquenil will likely provide sufficient benefit. If 40 to 60 mg/day is required for a response, the DMARD medications, such as azathioprine or methotrexate, will be needed to maintain the clinical benefit.

When prednisone of 5 mg or greater is used each day for longer than one month, a bisphosphonate (Fosamax 70 mg/week or Actonel 35 mg/

Steroid Doses and Risks

Low Dose: up to 7.5 mg per day
Low risk. This level is comparable to what is normally present in the body. These doses may be taken for many years with minimal side effects, which may be acceptable, depending upon the severity of the condition. The side effects that may occur with long-term use must be monitored.

Intermediate Dose: 7.5 to 20 mg per day
Modest risk. In the first month or so, the risk from this dosage is small. After this, risk increases, but many people still experience more benefit than risks.

High Dose: 20 to 60 mg per day
Higher risk in all cases. Corticosteroids at this dose have saved many lives and have prevented countless people from serious disease complications. Nevertheless, these amounts should only be used when clearly necessary because of the chance of side effects and serious problems. Dosage should be reduced, with the addition of other powerful anti-inflammmatory drugs, usually DMARDs, to help treat the disease.

Extremely High Dose: 100 to 1,000 mg per day
This dosage is used only in exceptional circumstances and only for the short term.

—Source: Arthritis Foundation

week) should also be taken to prevent steroid-induced osteoporosis. Also, a bone-density study should be obtained as a baseline and monitored at least yearly. Additional treatment may be necessary if the osteoporosis is or becomes severe. The status of prior exposure to tuberculosis should be established at the onset of steroid use because, even if patients have been exposed to tuberculosis (TB) they may no longer react to the skin test. In patients with a history of TB exposure either treated or not, a baseline chest X-ray is advisable. Some patients from certain countries outside the United States will have been vaccinated for TB, and they will have a positive test while never having had exposure to or infection by the actual TB organism.

It is also a good idea when starting immunomodulator therapy (a therapy that tones down the level of inflammation, such as methotrexate, azathioprine, and prednisone) to review your vaccination history. It may be a good idea to get hepatitis A and B vaccines or boosters if you had them but blood tests now show you no longer have protective immunity. Pneumovax, which protects against pneumococcal pneumonia, is recommended, with a booster approximately every six years. A "flu" vaccine is recommended yearly. And don't forget to check that tetanus booster recommended for every ten years or within five years if you've stepped on a rusty nail or received a cut with any exposure to soil.

Disease-Modifying Antirheumatic Drugs (DMARDs)

DMARDs are generally used in serious cases of inflammation and are sometimes prescribed as steroid-sparing drugs to take while you taper down from high-dose steroids. As you supplement your therapy with DMARDs, you can reduce the steroid, helping to avoid their unpleasant side effects. DMARDs can have serious side effects, but these are dependent on the amount you take. The effects are usually reversible once you reduce the dose or stop taking the drug completely.

This group includes azathioprine (Imuran), mycophenolate mofetil (CellCept), methotrexate (Rheumatrex), cyclosporine (Sandimmune), and cyclophosphamide (Cytoxan), all of which interfere with immune function. All these agents inhibit overactive immune-system cells to a greater extent than other cells by blocking various pathways in DNA synthesis and cell-division pathways. Some, such as methotrexate, also have additional anti-inflammatory actions. Methotrexate increases a substance called *adenosine* at sites of inflammation, which blocks an inflammatory pathway.

DMARDs slow down or in some cases can even stop the progression of inflammatory disease. Physicians sometimes prescribe DMARDs in combination. When drugs come to market they are almost exclusively studied and approved by the FDA in the U.S. as single agents (monotherapy). However, in treating patients various combinations of therapies will be explored to maximize their benefit. There has been some evidence that combinations of lower doses of several medications will actually result in better efficacy with fewer side effects. The strategy of aggressively treating "flares" of the inflammation, followed by tapering off the medications, can provide effective treatment with less exposure to these groups of medications. This would be expected to minimize both the short- and long-term risks to the patient. These types of strategies are most often tailored to the individual and have not been rigorously studied in the clinical trial format.

If your doctor prescribes any of these DMARDs, discuss the side effects thoroughly and stay in touch as you remain on the drug. There are potentially serious side effects, such as a lowering of your defenses against disease, but often the results justify their use and minimize exposure to longer use of steroids

Tetracyclines

A few additional medications can be helpful in special circumstances when the more standard therapy, such as Plaquenil and anti-inflammatory medication, is not working or when it has resulted in unacceptable side effects. One option is in the class of tetracyclines, a group of weak antibiotics that also block a pathway of inflammation called *metalloproteinase*. Doxycycline or Minocin (minocycline) can block this pathway in joints and result in less joint pain. Doxycycline may be associated with fewer side effects, including drug-induced lupus and vasculitis, and so is preferred as a first choice. Usually, a clinical response is noted in two weeks, and often an initial trial of three months can provide improvement in the arthritis when other agents have not proven acceptable.

Colchicine

Colchicine, a medicine derived from the seeds and tubers of the autumn crocus, has been in the medical literature for a long time. It is used regularly in the treatment of gout and Familial Mediterranean Fever. It blocks inflammatory responses and can exert its anti-inflammatory effect on many different tissues. It may be indicated for other inflammatory conditions like SjS and neuropathies in some patients. Colchicine has been reported to interfere with the absorption of some nutrients. Although the research remains inconsistent, those taking colchicine who experience symptoms associated with the nervous system (neuropathies) should discuss with their doctors having their blood levels of vitamin B_{12} measured and B_{12} administered should a deficiency be diagnosed. If you are taking this drug it is advisable to also take a high-potency multivitamin/mineral to compensate for a possible lack of absorption of some nutrients.

Intravenous Gamma Globulin

Intravenous gamma globulin (IVIG), the intravenous infusion of gamma globulin, may find an occasional place in the treatment armamentarium. It is done on an out-patient basis and generally takes about three hours. If steroids and DMARDs fail or cannot be used, then IVIG can provide immunomodulation without increasing the risk of infection. Occasionally there is a role for this therapy in complicated cases, such as severe immune-mediated neuropathies and vasculitis. The main downside is that IVIG is made from pooled human serum, which may contain yet-to-be-discovered infectious organisms for which we currently have no test. Taking this risk if you are very young is not reasonable; however, it is important to note that IVIG is the treatment of choice for young children who have a form of vasculitis called *Kawasaki disease* (mucocutaneous lymph node syndrome). The second major problem with IVIG is the cost, which approximates $1,000 per infusion for medication alone.

Antidepressants

Finally, there may be a role for selective serotonin reuptake inhibitors (SSRIs), a group of antidepressants, but their role in SjS is primarily to manage chronic pain, associated depression, or secondary fibromyalgia. Although there is some evidence that they decrease cell-mediated immune responses, the effect is only short-lived, and with chronic administration this effect no longer occurs.

New Medications

There are a few new immune-specific medications that are being explored to treat SjS. There is a relatively new class of medications called TNF alpha (tumor necrois alpha) blockers that are FDA approved for treating rheumatoid arthritis and psoriatic arthritis. A few published reports have appeared using one of the TNF blockers, Remicade (infliximab). The clinical benefit was first seen at two weeks and maintained through the fourteen-week study. Remicade is given as an IV infusion (3 mg/kg) at zero, two, and six weeks. The cost of this biologic medication (human monoclonal antibody with some mouse protein that specifically binds the TNF cytokine) is also in the $1,000 per dose range for medication alone. The higher the dose needed, the higher the cost. A recent report from one research group suggests that infliximab restores normal aquaporin distribution in the salivary gland, which might explain some of its benefits, including improvement of oral and ocular dryness. Aquaporins are a family of water-specific membrane channel proteins that may play a role in the decrease in salivary and lacrimal gland secretions.

Another biologic medication in clinical development is interferon alpha, or INF alpha (Veldona), which is a replica of the naturally occurring form of this cytokine in our bodies. A completed safety (Phase II) study suggested that the use of 150 IU lozenges three times per day for twelve weeks improved salivary secretions and decreased dry-mouth complaints.

New information is developing with the drug Rituxan (an anti-CD20 monoclonal antibody), which has been approved for treating B-cell lymphomas. Several studies are showing efficacy in other B-cell–driven immune disorders such as lupus and some cases of rhuematoid arthritis.

Some of these drugs have been approved for use with other conditions. If they sound useful to you, any of these off-label indications should be discussed in detail with your rheumatologist.

Keeping Track of Your Medications

Finally, whatever medication you choose, make sure you keep a complete list and the amount of your dose. A helpful tool for keeping track of your medications is to keep a chart. Having a list of medications, the prescribing doctor, and whether you found the medications agreed with you or not helps in the overall management of your disorder. Here is a template that you may use, one we have found helpful. You may want to make two lists: the first will represent the drugs you currently use, and the second will outline your history of drugs taken but perhaps discontinued. Medications can play an important role in the management of Sjögren's syndrome. Being an informed patient will help you make the choices that will make your road a little smoother.

A Medic-Alert bracelet becomes a necessity when taking any of these drugs. Wearing the bracelet at all times assures you that you will not be given a medication in an emergency situation that would conflict with those that your body has come to depend on and that important information will always be available to emergency medical personnel. Once you register with Medic-Alert, they will have a complete list of your medications on file and will respond immediately to any call for information. At a reasonable cost, you will be well protected.

Date Started	Drug + Amount	Prescribing Physician	Reason	Date Stopped	Comments

11

Nutrition and
Autoimmune Disorders

BALANCED NUTRITION, THE FULL COMPLEMENT
of nutrients in proper amounts for health, is necessary for everyone and
particularly for anyone suffering from an autoimmune disorder. Without
a full complement of nutrients, we cannot survive. And, with less than a
full complement, the body cannot effectively heal itself. Our need for nutrients varies with the ever-changing needs of our bodies. These needs are
affected by age, gender, body size, and the presence of certain disease conditions. Chronic and infectious diseases place a wide range of physiologi-
cal stresses on our bodies that require nutritional adjustments to manage.
In this chapter, we will focus on the interrelationships of nutrition and the
immune system, particularly for the purpose of the management of autoimmune disorders, including SjS.

While it is optimal to get all your nutrients from the foods you eat,
supplements are often necessary. Your rheumatologist may have specific
recommendations on how you can better balance your nutrition. Many dietary adjustments will be lifelong commitments in order to effectively treat
SjS. If supplementation is required, its effects will need to be monitored
closely by a physician.

Necessary Nutrients

Our bodies need nutrients, including carbohydrates, fats, and proteins, in relatively large amounts for energy. In addition to providing energy, the components of these carbohydrates, fats, and proteins are indispensable in the regulation of the activity of enzymes and hormones, and in the function of the immune and the nervous systems. Other nutrients, vitamins, minerals, and trace elements also play a crucial role in the management and regulation of all these vital functions.

There are nearly fifty nutrients that are all needed to function in concert to sustain life. The amounts required and the timing of their presence in specific cells and organs are regulated through highly sophisticated mechanisms. We cannot afford to have the supply of any nutrient drop below critical levels. Therein lies the importance of maintaining adequate nutrition for health.

While most of our nutritional needs come from the foods we eat, many people rely on nutritional supplements to augment or ensure their intakes of nutrients. It is possible to confuse nutritional supplements, such as vitamins, minerals, and omega-3 fatty acids, with dietary supplements, which go beyond nutrients to include herbs and other botanicals. This is a very confusing and potentially dangerous situation. The Food and Drug Administration does not regulate the safety and efficacy of dietary supple-

---

Essential Nutrients

Water

Sources of energy: Carbohydrates, fats, and proteins in amounts to meet our energy needs

Essential amino acids: lysine, methionine, threonine, tryptophan, leucine, isoleucine, phenylalanine, histidine, valine

Essential fatty acids: linoleic acid, linolenic acid, eicosapentaenoic acid (EPA), and docosahexaenoic acid (DHA)

Minerals: calcium, phosphorus, iron, sodium, potassium, chlorine, fluorine, iodine, sulfur, magnesium, manganese, copper, cobalt, chromium, molybdenum, zinc, selenium, vanadium, nickel, silicon, tin, boron

Vitamins: retinol (vitamin A), thiamin (B_1), riboflavin (B_2), niacin (B_3), pyridoxine (B_6), pantothenic acid, biotin, folic acid, cyanocobalamin (B_{12}), ascorbate (C), calciferol (D), tocopherol (E)

ments. In most cases, we do not know what good or harm these herbs and botanicals might do to us. So, for safety's sake, we will only concern ourselves with nutrients that have been studied and proven beneficial. For further information on complementary medicine, see Chapter 12.

It is necessary for everyone to eat a nutritionally balanced diet to ensure a healthy immune system. That goes for all of us, whether or not we suffer from an autoimmune disease. As a Sjögren's syndrome sufferer, you may have to make adjustments to your eating pattern, without compromising your balanced diet. For example, you may become discouraged from eating dry foods like crackers and pretzels in favor of soft bread and muffins. You may have to favor soft, less chewy foods also because the lack of saliva leads to serious problems with tooth decay.

You may need to avoid large meals in favor of small, more frequent meals to accommodate any gastrointestinal inflammation discomfort or motility problems. Well-planned small meals deliver the same nutrients as larger less frequent ones. One way of achieving this change without adding extra calories is to borrow from your breakfast, lunch, or dinner some foods that you can eat in the in-between meals. These practices should not compromise the nutritional quality of the diet.

A Guide to a Nutritionally Balanced Diet		
Food Group	**Daily Servings***	**Recommended Choices**
Bread, Cereal, Rice, Pasta	6–11**	A wide variety of whole grains and wheat germ, with no added sugar or fat
Fruits & Vegetables	5–10	Dark green, leafy, and cruciferous vegetables; berries; citrus; pears; and melons
Milk, Yogurt & Cheese	2–3**	Soy milk and soy products; nonfat and unsweetened products
Meat, Poultry, Fish, Dry Beans, Eggs & Nuts	2–3**	Oily fish; limit eggs with no fat added to 2–3 per week and lean red meat to 1–2 times per week
Fats, Oils & Sweets	Sparingly	Restrict to soy, canola, or olive oils. Avoid sweets and added sugar.

*Always adjust selection, serving, and meal sizes to comfortable digestion.

** Serving sizes are stated on the Nutrition Facts label of most foods. If you have weight problems reduce the serving size of all foods, except for beans, fruits, and vegetables.

—Information modified from the USDA Pyramid Food Guide (*www.nutrition.gov*).

How Nutrition Helps Manage Autoimmunity

The role of nutrition in the management of autoimmune diseases takes on many forms. Some of them seem unrelated. This is primarily attributed to the wide variety of symptoms and the rather sketchy understanding of the metabolic events associated with autoimmune diseases. Dr. Sjögren merely described the symptoms and suggested that they represented a clinical entity worthy of investigation. We have come a long way toward understanding the conditions under which these symptoms tend to develop. We are progressing toward identifying related clinical symptoms and blood tests that will eventually shed more light on the nutritional needs of patients.

As we have said, the immune system mistakenly attacks one's own tissues and may cause inflammation in autoimmune conditions. Autoimmunity and inflammation bring about a variety of metabolic changes that impact many of the body's functions. Among those changes are hormones, especially cortisone, insulin, and thyroxin, that become less effective. Cortisone becomes elevated in response to stress conditions and results in the disturbance of mineral metabolism and water retention. Insulin regulates carbohydrate metabolism and fat storage. Thyroxin controls body temperature and energy utilization. Autoimmune events involve many tissues and organs as well as the immune and the central nervous systems. This is a systemic reaction occurring throughout the body, not a contained trauma.

In this chapter you will learn how nutritional support through diet and supplements can decrease the inflammatory responses associated with autoimmunity. You will also learn how proper nutrition can help manage the side effects of some of the medications frequently used to treat SjS.

We should bear in mind that, at present, nutrition in autoimmunity is a dynamic area of study. New information is being generated and tested in many research institutions all the time. It is likely that we will see an extension of our current nutrition knowledge in ways that will make it possible to more effectively manage many of the troubling symptoms.

The Importance of Fat

Inflammation, and therefore the symptoms with which it is associated, is common to other diseases, including heart disease, obesity, and diabetes.

Six Dietary Recommendations for Autoimmune Disease

1. Avoid animal fat, except for oily fish.
2. Favor a predominantly vegetarian diet.
3. Consume whole grains, fruits, and vegetables that are rich in vitamins E and C, especially bright-colored ones, such as broccoli, red and green sweet peppers, and spinach.
4. When adding oils to foods, use canola, soy, safflower, sunflower, and olive oils.
5. Take a well-balanced all-inclusive vitamin and mineral supplement that includes 100 percent of the RDA for each of the vitamins and minerals.
6. If advised by your rheumatologist, look for an antioxidant supplement containing vitamin E and C, carotenoids, and selenium; a bone-strengthening supplement containing calcium, magnesium, and vitamin D; an omega-3 fatty acids supplement containing EPA, DHA, and vitamin E; and a B-vitamin supplement that is particularly rich in vitamin B_6, folic acid, and vitamin B_{12}.

In all of these conditions, fat plays a major role. However, our view of fat has been off the mark.

Nutritionists are now raising awareness of the fact that the condemnation and trivialization of fat has been unfounded. Obsessed with thinness, we have rushed to eliminate fat from our diets. Fearful of heart disease, we have sought foods low in fat and cholesterol. Concerned about diabetes, we have tried ways to reduce carbohydrates as well. This panic has created serious confusion about ideal dietary practices and often has led many of us to try extreme diets, not always with the health benefits we sought. The important concept to emphasize here is that fats and oils are not equal in their harmful effects or nutritional benefits. Our strategy should not be to reduce or eliminate fat as much as to limit our consumption of fat to that which is of high nutritional quality.

UNSATURATED FAT

Fats are made up of individual fatty acids strung together in threes. Most of these fatty acids are long straight chains. One end of the chain is acidic and soluble in water, while the rest of the molecule is soluble in fatty material. If the fatty acids lose hydrogen, they become unsaturated. This unsaturation may occur in several places along the fatty-acid molecule, giving rise to polyunsaturated fatty acids. When carbon 6 is unsaturated, the fatty acid is called omega-6; when carbon 3 is unsaturated, it is called omega-3 fatty acid. These unsaturated fatty acids, found predominantly in oils, tend to fold onto themselves rather than lie flat and straight like the saturated fats, which are found mainly in hard fats like butter, shortenings, some margarines, and lard. The natural folded form is called *cis,* and must be distinguished from the unfolded unsaturated fatty acids, called *trans.*

Diets high in saturated and *trans*–fatty acids raise our blood cholesterol, but nutritionists remind us that rather than strive to eliminate fat from our diets, we need to achieve a balance of the types of fats and oils we consume. It has long been recognized that the more unsaturated fat we eat, the lower our blood cholesterol will be. Our bodies can easily make all the saturated fatty acids we need. So, instead of consuming saturated fat it is important to concentrate on consuming a variety of oils that would supply a mixture of the omega-6 and the omega-3 fatty acids in the natural *cis* form.

ESSENTIAL FATTY ACIDS

There is more to polyunsaturated fatty acids (PUFA) than lowering our blood cholesterol and protecting our hearts. Omega-6 (linoleic) and omega-3 (linolenic, eicosapentenoic [EPA], and docosahexaenoic [DHA]) fatty acids are PUFAs that are considered essential nutrients. You may recognize these tongue-twister names from labels of nutritional supplements.

One important function of essential fatty acids is to form an integral part of the cell membrane, which regulates what goes in and out of the cells and anchors molecules to the cell surface. It is possible that fatty acids have an effect on the function of some of the molecules imbedded in the cell membrane that are recognized by the immune system and thus are termed *antigens.* Like the functions of many nutrients, those of fats are subject to checks and balances.

Omega-6 Fatty Acids

Our bodies have the capacity to produce saturated fatty acids and to store them as energy reserves in fat tissue. Our bodies can also desaturate these fatty acids, turning them into omega-6 fatty acids, with the exception of one—linoleic acid. Since we cannot produce it in our tissue and because it is an essential nutrient, linoleic acid must be obtained from food. An important function of linoleic acid, an essential fatty acid, is that it forms arachidonic acid, which in turn forms eicosanoids. These compounds are described in the scientific literature as *lipid mediators*. They regulate the function of the lipids (fatty compounds) inside and outside the cell. Linoleic acid is found in corn oil, sunflower oil, and safflower oil. To integrate these oils into your diet, use them instead of saturated fat sources such as butter or hydrogenated oil. Most important, however, is keeping a healthy balance of omega-6s and omega-3s (see the omega-3 section below) in your diet to fight against inflammatory symptoms of SjS.

Omega-3 Fatty Acids

While some seed oils, especially canola, contain omega-3 fatty acids, they are most abundant in fish oils. It has been known for some time that consuming oily fish rich in omega-3 fatty acids reduces the incidence of cardiovascular diseases. But research has shown that omega-3s can also reduce the occurrence of symptoms associated with SjS.

Omega-3 fatty acids act to regulate the amount and the timing of the release of the eicosanoids—lipid regulators (including prostaglandins, leukotrienes, and thromboxanes) formed from arachidonic acid. The check-and-balance system omega-3s provide for the production of eicosanoids is extremely important as they should only be produced when needed and in precisely the right amounts. We know that an increased formation of eicosanoids coincides with flares of autoimmune disorders. We also know that high intake of omega-3 fatty acids over a long period of time curbs the overproduction of eicosanoids, and this adjustment improves the symptoms of a variety of autoimmune diseases, including SjS.

To increase the amount of omega-3s in your diet, incorporate oily fish such as salmon, mackerel, sardines, eel, and sablefish, also called Pacific black cod, into your meals. Try to incorporate these fish into your meals once or twice a week. Linolenic acid is also found in soybean and canola oils. The diet of Greenland Eskimos, which includes 6 to 10 grams of EPA and DHA a day, is considered to be the reason that the occurrence of rheumatoid arthritis in their population is less severe than in populations that eat fish less than once a week. Fish oils are also available as a supplement.

You can choose to take fish-oil supplements in order to get more omega-3 fatty acids into your diet. In one study on rheumatoid arthritic patients the beneficial effect of a lacto-vegetarian-fish oil–supplemented diet was confirmed within two months. If a supplement of fish oil is needed to ameliorate inflammation associated with autoimmunity look for capsules containing 1 to 2 grams of EPA and DHA. You may go higher on the advice of your rheumatologist as long as you do not develop side effects, such as diarrhea. For those with autoimmune conditions, dosage requirements will differ from person to person and vary in response to the progress of the disease and interaction with specific medications.

Because fish oils in supplement form are subject to oxidation when refined, choose only those containing vitamin E as an antioxidant and only buy preparations that are stored in a refrigerator. Oily fish itself is not subject to a refining process and therefore contains enough vitamin E to preserve the unsaturated fatty acids. Oxidation could result in molecular changes and the disturbance of the composition of cell membranes, which in itself could trigger autoimmune flares. You should also protect your cells by adding antioxidants such as vitamins C and E and selenium to your diet. Furthermore, antioxidant vitamins have been shown to slow the liberation of arachidonic acid and the formation of eicosanoid compounds, which are associated with the triggering of flares of inflammation in patients with autoimmune diseases.

Note: Flaxseed oil capsules are often promoted as a source of omega-3 fatty acids. While this may be true, many nutritionists are doubtful of the wisdom of consuming flaxseed oil for safety reasons. We therefore focus our attention on oily fish and fish-oil supplements. While we are on the issue of safety, we should point out that because of contamination with polychlorinated biphenyls (PCB), methyl mercury, and other pollutants in certain fish, pregnant and nursing women, or those planning pregnancy within a year, are advised against eating bluefish, striped bass, swordfish, shark, king mackerel, tuna steaks, white and golden snapper, and any freshwater fish. Canned tuna should be limited to 5 ounces a week.

Facts about Fats		
Sources of Fats*	**Main Sources**	**Value to Inflammation/ Autoimmunity**
Monounsaturated Fatty Acids	Canola and olive oils and their products	Moderate: Lowers LDL and total cholesterol.
Polyunsaturated Fatty Acids (PUFA)	Canola, soy, safflower, sunflower and corn, contain mainly omega-6 and some omega-3 while fish oils and their products contain mostly omega-3	Valuable: Lowers LDL and total cholesterol.
Saturated Fatty Acids	Animal fat from meat, milk, and butter	Negative: Raises LDL and total cholesterol.
Trans–Fatty Acids	Partially hydrogenated vegetable oils used in cooking oils, margarine, and commercially baked and fried foods.	Negative: Raises LDL and total cholesterol.

*NOTE: Fats are solid and oils are fluid at room temperature. Fats tend to be high in saturated fatty acids, whereas oils contain more unsaturated fatty acids. Tropical vegetable oils, such as palm and coconut oils, are the exception in that they are high in saturated fatty acids.

The Protective Nutrients

SELENIUM

We mentioned selenium as an antioxidant that protects PUFA and the integrity of cell membranes. It should be recognized that selenium, copper, and zinc share the same transporting protein for their absorption in the intestines. So, it is best to separate a selenium supplement from a multimineral supplement by about two hours. These minerals are components of metalloproteins, the formation of which is stimulated under some autoimmune conditions, like rheumatic diseases. This may result in increased storage of iron and zinc in the liver, while not making them available to peripheral tissues, which may result in the anemic symptoms sometimes associated with autoimmune diseases. For this reason, a multimineral supplement is often recommended. Commonly, daily intakes of 50 mcg selenium, 15 mg zinc, 2 mg copper, and 10 mg iron are recommended.

VITAMIN B$_{12}$ AND FOLIC ACID

Vitamin B$_{12}$ and folic acid are needed for the formation of glutathione, which is part of the antioxidation process. These two nutrients have to be in balance; taking folic acid as a supplement may mask the deficiency symptoms of vitamin B$_{12}$. Also one complication of autoimmunity might be the development of type A gastritis, which is the thinning of the gastric (stomach) mucosa and the loss of the gastric mucosal fold, which is often related to malabsorption of vitamin B$_{12}$. Low blood levels of vitamin B$_{12}$ result in the development of pernicious anemia. Often, a supplement of up to 100 mcg of vitamin B$_{12}$ and 400 mcg of folic acid may be recommended.

Nutrition Management of Medications

If you require prednisone or a similar therapy to treat SjS or other auto-immune conditions, you will need to protect the density of your bone with additional calcium, magnesium, and vitamin D, along with a larger intake of protein and increased weight-bearing exercises. Your doctor will have you monitor your bone-density levels and suggest the appropriate supplements as well as bisphosphonate medications. Treatment with prednisone will increase your susceptibility to infections and thus will require your extreme diligence to avoid anyone with an infectious disease.

While we suspect that there are possibly other drug-nutrient interactions, there are few hard data at this time. In an earlier chapter we mentioned the need for an assessment of vitamin B$_{12}$ when taking colchicine. There is evidence that this drug interferes with the absorption of this B vitamin. Other interactions are not so clear. Consider, with your doctor, pharmacist, and nutritionist, whether your medications may be interfering with your nutrient availability, and adjust amounts and timing to optimize their effects.

Complementary Medicine

SJÖGREN'S SYNDROME (SjS) IS A CHRONIC, ONGO-
ing disorder; there is no magic bullet (yet) to eradicate its symptoms. There
is no medication or treatment available at this time that will prevent the
"flares." Still, there are things patients can do to help make the flares less
stressful; many of them fall under the purview of complementary or alternative medicine.

Just as flying an airplane relies on multiple strategies for success, so too
does managing this syndrome. With you as pilot, conventional medicine
as copilot, and complementary medicine as navigator, it is possible for
your body to come in for a soft landing. It takes a balance of conventional
medical diagnosis and treatment with mind/body/spirit techniques to
manage a chronic disease like SjS.

Complementary or *alternative medicine* is defined as a group of diverse
medical and health-care systems, practices, and products that are not currently considered part of conventional medicine. Conventional medicine
is that practiced by holders of an M.D. (Doctor of Medicine) or O.D.
(Doctor of Osteopathy) and by allied practitioners such as physical therapists, nurses, dietitians, art therapists, and psychologists. Other terms for
conventional medicine are *allopathy, Western medicine, mainstream medicine,* and *traditional medicine.* Complementary medicine techniques—
meditation, massage therapy, movement therapy, biofeedback—begin

with the belief that wellness is based on the body's return to balance using its own energy force and wisdom to heal and remain well. Complementary medicine can be used together with conventional medicine.

When complementary medicine is used in conjunction with conventional medicine, the emphasis shifts from the standpoint of fixing a diseased body part to that of healing the whole person—body, mind, and spirit. The new terminology for this blended medical treatment is *integrative medicine* and, increasingly, at medical centers in large urban areas, you can find centers of integrative medicine where both conventional and complementary or alternative medicine practitioners work hand in hand. Physicians, skilled in both types of medical care can be found treating patients. The practitioner and patient work together to bring the body's innate healing capacity into play. Again, the concept of partnership is more effective in treating these disorders.

What Is Integrative Medicine?

Integrative medicine is an individualized combination of conventional and complementary treatments that is used to restore balance to the patient's mind, body, and spirit. While you incorporate mind-body systems such as body movement, meditation, visualization, and biofeedback, you will continue to utilize modern diagnostic and treatment techniques available through conventional medicine. Because complementary medicine can help manage pain, reduce your reliance on medication, and help overcome the side effects of many treatments, integrative treatments may enable you to cut back on your traditional medications.

Is Integrative Medicine Safe?

Since the early 1990s when alternative medicine entered the mainstream, research into its use and practice has gained momentum. In 1992, the National Institutes of Health (NIH) created an Office of Alternative Medicine with a $2-million budget; in 1998 it became the National Center for Complementary and Alternative Medicine, with a current budget of $100 million, and the amount allocated for 2003 is $111 million.

Between 1990 and 1997, visits to complementary medicine providers in the United States increased 47 percent to 625 million. Today, half of all adults use such treatments. In a study of 831 adults published in 2001, it was reported that of those who saw a medical doctor and concurrently used complementary therapies in the previous twelve months, 79 percent perceived the combination to be superior to either one alone. Of 411 respondents who reported seeing both a medical doctor and a complementary provider, 70 percent typically saw a medical doctor before or concurrent with their visits to a complementary provider, and perceived confidence in complementary providers was not substantially different from confidence in medical doctors. Interestingly, of the 831 respondents who in the past year had used a complementary therapy and seen a medical doctor, 63 to 72 percent did not disclose at least one type of complementary therapy to the medical doctor.

Does this mean that patients are rejecting conventional medicine for alternative strategies? No, the data do not support this. Rather it appears that those who use the integrative approach appear to value both and tend to be less concerned about their medical doctor's disapproval than about his or her inability to understand or incorporate complementary medical diagnoses and treatments into their medical management. If your doctor is unwilling to work in partnership with you and the rest of your team, it may be time to find a new provider or to encourage your doctor to take a look at this concept of healing.

However, the fact that 63 to 72 percent of those using complementary healing techniques did not inform their doctor is worrying. ALWAYS consult with your physician so that she can advise and guide you and oversee the effects of all of your treatments. Bring a list and description of all your herbal preparations.

THE PLACEBO EFFECT

Study after study has shown that while the medical community has questioned the validity of certain complementary techniques, objective reports demonstrate that, at the very least, acupuncture, biofeedback, massage, and meditation reduce chronic pain. The doubters tend to dismiss this phenomenon as the "placebo" effect, where the patient may become psychologically convinced of the relief of pain. This should not negate the fact that these treatments do relieve pain.

LEARNING MORE ABOUT INTEGRATIVE MEDICINE

Perhaps you are curious about whether or not these treatments will work for you. It's good to be curious and a bit skeptical. There are well over 300 different types of practice lumped into the category of complementary medicine, everything from healing with crystals to medically endorsed practices such as biofeedback and yoga. Your job is to find the ones that you feel would be the most helpful to you. This can be confusing but not impossible. If you are considering complementary medicine, here are five steps to take:

- Do your research first. Read about the treatment, ask friends who have used it, search the web for information, and be wary of anything that makes claims to "cure" your disorder. Claims are enticing but most often misleading and false.
- Check with your physician for its applicability in your case. Make sure it does no harm.
- Ask your physician for names and suggestions of clinics.
- Check the credentials to make certain that the practitioner has been properly trained and licensed if licensure is available in your state.
- Try one session first.

A good place to begin your research is with the Arthritis Foundation's book *A Guide to Alternative Therapies,* written by Judith Horstman. It is an official publication of the Arthritis Foundation and can be purchased through their web site or by telephone. It describes the meaning of each alternative healing system (Ayurvedic, Chinese, osteopathic, and chiropractic medicine), clarifies the differences among the many types of body work, and then goes on to discuss the various herbs and remedies offered as curatives. It is a responsible and comprehensive assessment of what alternative (we prefer to call it complementary) medicine has to offer.

In an earlier chapter we mentioned a book that has a comprehensive easy-to-read description of the science of integrative medicine as well as descriptions of each of the modalities available. The author has set aside a special chapter to deal with specific problems such as joint and muscle pain, headache, fibromyalgia, and dental pain. James N. Dillard, M.D., D.C., C.Ac. (diplomas in medicine, chiropractic, and acupuncture), is assistant clinical professor, Columbia University College of Physicians and

Surgeons and clinical advisor to Columbia's Rosenthal Center for Complementary and Alternative Medicine. His book is *The Chronic Pain Solution* (New York: Bantam, 2002).

A quick search on the Internet will also reap great rewards. We have listed several informative web sites on pages 171–72. The best place to begin is the American Holistic Medical Association (AHMA), where you can locate a doctor in your area to assist you in your search. Another excellent resource is the National Center for Complementary and Alternative Medicine (NCCAM) at the National Institutes of Health. This government department posts guidelines for choosing an alternative practitioner on their web site as well as the latest news about complementary and alternative medicine from their research.

Once you have an understanding of the various options available to you, take your ideas to your doctor. Together, work out a plan for integrating your health care with her. Perhaps she is knowledgeable about these practices and knows of good practitioners. Have her refer you to these centers. Then check the accreditation of the practitioner. Not all states require licensure of practitioners, but the national boards can provide you with guidelines when shopping for a specialist. We list some of the professional associations in the Resource section at the end of this book. Many health plans cover some of the treatments.

Alternative Treatment Options

There are many types of practice lumped into the category of alternative or complementary medicine. Your job is to find the ones that you need. We can't possibly list every one but there are some that work better than others for the specific problems associated with SjS.

Below is a list of some of the most useful alternative treatments for SjS patients. Some patients will benefit from other techniques, depending upon what part of the body is primarily affected. For example, if you have Raynaud's disease along with SjS, you may find massage, acupuncture, and qi gong helpful. If you suffer from unknown food allergies, the elimination diet may help identify your triggers. Since this book cannot be exhaustive in its presentation, please look further and talk to your doctor about treatments that could be right for you.

MASSAGE THERAPY

Massage therapy is part of a group of alternative medical systems called *manipulative and body-based methods* that are based on the manipulation or movement of one or more parts of the body. Massage allows you to relax in a warm and soothing environment, *keep your eyes closed,* drift off, and allow your muscles to relax under the skilled hands of a massage therapist. You lie facedown with your eyes soothingly closed on a table covered with a blanket in a warm room while a massage therapist gently massages painful muscles and joints. Eileen's massage therapist places a warm water-filled cushion on the table for her to lie on. Every once in a while Darlene treats herself to a "hot stone" massage during which the therapist massages her body with stones that have been heated first and then immersed in almond oil before application to her tired muscles. While this may not suit you, allowing your body to enjoy a regular massage is one of the gifts you can give yourself. There are different kinds of massage, each of which is described in the books referred to earlier. Check the accreditation of your practitioner by asking her, or check through the National Certification Board for Therapeutic Massage and Bodywork.

YOGA

An ancient system of body/mind/spirit meditation and movement, yoga focuses your attention on your body to gently restore it to harmony. Yoga includes meditation, gentle stretches, and balancing exercises. It can help you relax and ease your pain by focusing your attention on your breathing while moving your body. Yoga lifts depression and increases circulation, strength, flexibility, and balance. Study the various types of yoga that are offered. Those with SjS will benefit from a form of yoga, such as hatha yoga, that is slow and gentle enough to respond to the body's suggestion. Make sure that this will do for you what you want. Speak to the teacher and explain what you wish to heal before joining the class. Ask if she has experience working with impaired mobility and chronic pain. There are many books that you will find at your library and Internet sources for information on yoga.

QI GONG

Qi gong (chee kung) is an ancient Chinese form of meditation and movement that you may find to be gentler than others. Meditation and breathing are the centerpiece; gentle movement holds your body in balance. This practice can be done sitting down if you are uncomfortable standing. Those with SjS will respond to the gentle massages of eyes, head, and glands. If you have difficulty locating a qi gong class in your neighborhood, check with the physiotherapists or health centers nearby. We found ours at a nearby senior center. Check the Internet for qi gong web sites and the local libraries for videos and books describing this age-old healing technique.

MEDITATION

Meditation has roots in our earliest religions from Christianity to Zen Buddhism. It is a way of quieting our minds to reduce the stress in our bodies and emotions. Scientific studies have shown that practicing mindfulness meditation benefits those living with chronic pain and illness. Specifically, research has demonstrated that mindfulness meditation decreases pain and physical symptoms by 30 percent and decreases depression, anxiety, and anger by 60 percent. Most important, these studies have found that those who practice mindfulness find their lives to be fulfilling and peaceful regardless of their circumstances.

Mindfulness meditation may be a new phrase for you. It means simply that you pay attention to the present moment. Doing so can be profound; the present moment is where our lives unfold, where our tenderness and strength reside, and where choice is possible. Mindfulness is subtle and powerful. It moves into your life and the world. It can inform your interactions at home, on the freeway, in the supermarket, and at work. The practice of mindfulness asks that we cultivate compassion for ourselves and others as we move through life.

If you would like to discover mindfulness, try this meditation. It was given to us by Amy Saltzman, M.D., of Palo Alto, California. Her clinic, For Yourself: Health, is an example of the blend of East-West medicine that we discuss in this chapter. You may read the following paragraph and then give it a try. Take your time and go slow.

A Brief Sitting Meditation

Meditation is a time for yourself, a time to return to the present moment. Begin by attending to your breath, the natural cycle of expansion, stillness, contraction, and stillness. As you inhale and exhale, allow the breath to fill you and empty you, empty you and fill you.

As you clear your thoughts, keep your attention focused on your breath and begin to attend to your senses. Be curious and compassionate about your experience in this moment. Explore the subtleties and complexities of sensation. Expand your attention to include sound. Listen with your entire being. Allow the next sound to call you home to the present moment.

Anchor yourself in the breath and begin to attend to your thoughts; simply observing your thoughts, without believing them or taking them personally. Focus your attention on whatever aspect of your experience is most prominent: breath, sensation, sound, thought, emotion. Meet your experience with an open heart. Now allow the phenomena of your experience to recede and rest in the spaces of stillness and peace.

Do this for an increasing period of time. Many people allocate time each day to seek silence, calm their breath, and meditate.

BIOFEEDBACK

Biofeedback is part of a group of practices that use a variety of techniques to enhance the mind's capacity to affect bodily function and symptoms. Also in this category are prayer, music and dance, meditation, and support groups. Biofeedback is meditation plus technology. If you find it difficult to meditate but would like to experience its benefits, ask your physician to refer you to a certified biofeedback operator. The operator instructs you in breathing and calming techniques. Using an electronic device to measure your skin temperature, electrical impulses from your muscles, and your heart rate, you will actually see the electronic scale change as you become calm through the techniques you use. The visual effect of seeing the readings go down is a powerful one. Soon, you will be able to do this by yourself. It is an excellent way to reduce pain in your muscles and joints, and cold in your extremities. Check with your doctor for a qualified biofeedback operator. Often they can be found in your local hospital.

A WORD OF CAUTION

Complementary medicine suffers, as do most new things, from haphazard regulations and claims. Anyone can claim anything for an herbal product or activity as long as he does not declare that it cures disease! For example, a product or technique may not say "will cure arthritis" but can proclaim "Thousands agree! Joint relief in ten days!" So buyer beware; check the technique and check the practitioner before putting your body at risk. And then remember that something that works for your neighbor may not be good for you. Begin slowly and assess your body after each session. The techniques mentioned here are safe and noninvasive. Others may be effective, or not, depending upon who you are and what the treatment is.

If you are tempted by herbs, vitamins, or other "natural" remedies, check out the excellent brochure published by the Arthritis Foundation described on page 172.

These warnings aside, great benefits can be had by combining Eastern and Western medicine. Balance is attainable, and pleasure in using your body is the reward.

Support Groups

The SjS Foundation publishes a monthly newsletter with information, research, and answers to questions. Through them, you can locate a contact person who will help answer any specific questions you may have. They also run small, supportive gatherings in which others with SjS can discuss treatments, doctors, diagnoses, and helpful tips for day-to-day living. Often these groups will have special speakers. Many of them have been established for several years, and members have become friends.

You can get from each meeting as much as you need: a tip here or there, a friend to call when things get bad, or simply a phone list so you can ask questions when they arise. We heartily recommend that you call and see if you might enjoy a meeting. If driving is a problem, ask if another member can drive. Some people stay away from support groups because they fear that the experience may be depressing. If this is how you feel and you have questions about SjS, call the leader to learn more about the syndrome and the way in which the group operates. She may provide the support you need on the telephone. But be encouraged, because with support, attention to your body, and some meditative and exercise techniques, you and your SjS will become harmonious.

Afterword

As this book goes to press, the mystery of Sjögren's syndrome is being unraveled. New diagnostic techniques, tests, and treatments that were not available when we began work on this book have been discovered. They hold great promise. By the time our book arrives on the shelves, these discoveries and others will continue to fuel our hope.

Thanks to the lobbying efforts of the Sjögren's Syndrome Foundation in the United States, similar groups in other countries, and scientists everywhere, awareness of the disorder has increased. Those of us with Sjögren's syndrome may not need to suffer in the future.

Researchers in Toronto have made a breakthrough discovery of a possible vaccine for SjS. Reported in the October 5, 2002, issue of *The Lancet*, they describe using a mouse model that naturally develops SjS on which they were able to identify a protein (ICA69) that is a major target in the autoimmune response that results in SjS. They developed a prototype vaccine to treat the condition. It dramatically reduced the tissue damage even relatively late in the animal model. Even after the disease had been operative, they were able to reverse the disease activity. These are encouraging, even exciting, results that could possibly mean the eradication of the disorder, at least in some individuals.

There are new technologies for autoimmune testing. Scientists at Stanford University have developed new antigen microarrays that will make diagnosis possible "on the spot" and facilitate patient screening. It will not be necessary to wait for weeks for blood work to return and be analyzed; results will be more conclusive on the initial doctor's visit. This same test may make it possible to predict who will develop SjS.

There is further optimism on the treatment front involving a therapy that has already been approved for rheumatoid arthritis, TNF blocker infliximab. In a one-year extension of a study of sixteen primary Sjögren's syndrome patients, ten patients received an infusion of infliximab (Remicade, 3 to 5 mg/kg) about every twelve weeks. Some improvement in eye and mouth symptoms as well as fatigue was seen. Perhaps most interesting is that a few of the patients from the initial study were considered to be in remission, and no additional infusions were given during the one-year extension study.

These and future exciting discoveries hold great hope for the future. As we now look to the ultimate conquest of this disorder, we have every reason to be optimistic. Anyone suffering with chronic disease knows that it is better to live with optimism than with pessimism. While patients didn't ask to get sick and they don't like being sick, they can glean some benefit from the condition. Chronic disease causes us to consider our lives in ways we did not have to before. We learn to count our blessings, and, perhaps as newly created optimists, we find "silver linings" that we weren't even aware of before. We learn to accentuate the positive: the beauty of a day, the silence of a moment, the blessing of a friend, the hug of a family member. Perhaps we learn different ways of thinking that add value to our lives that we never thought possible. And in case you think we overemphasize optimism, remember that there have been studies to show the positive effect of optimism on health.

So, where do we go from here? Decrease stress, eat nutritious foods, and exercise. But most important, hold on to the idea that you are not your disease; it does not control you. The disease hampers everyone who suffers with it, of course. But with optimism, a joyful view of the future, balance, good friends, and a strong partnership and respectful relationship between doctor and patient, life with Sjögren's syndrome can be rich and fulfilling.

Remember the epigraph of the book? It is as true today as when Hillel wrote it, that no matter what adversaries block our paths, we keep searching and living life as fully as we can. ". . . Meanwhile, I keep dancing."

Let's keep on dancing as together we head down the promising road toward a complete eradication of Sjögren's syndrome.

Appendix

Clinical Guidelines for Oral Treatment and Dental Caries Prevention in Patients with Chronic Dry Mouth

Troy Daniels, D.D.S., M.S.; Ava Wu, D.D.S.;
and Ernest Newbrun, D.M.D., Ph.D.
School of Dentistry, University of California
San Francisco, California

These guidelines are primarily for use by health-care professionals providing oral treatment and dental caries prevention for their patients with chronic hyposalivation due to Sjögren's syndrome, past head and neck radiation therapy, chronic use of drugs impairing salivary secretion, or other causes. The guidelines may also be useful to help affected patients better understand the often complex treatment that may be necessary. Some of these procedures can be performed only by dentists or dental hygienists. *Note:* The authors do not endorse any product in these guidelines. Brand names of products are used when a generic description would be inadequate or when branded products are the only ones available.

Dental Caries Prevention and Treatment

DIET

Each patient needs to be taught the role of dietary sugars in dental caries development and the need to confine sugar intake to meals and eliminate sugar between meals. Recommend *sugar-free* (but *not sugarless*) beverages, gum, etc., containing noncariogenic sweetening agents: for example, xylitol, sorbitol, saccharin (Sweet'n Low), aspartame (NutraSweet), or sucralose (Splenda).

ORAL HYGIENE

Each patient needs to be taught how to effectively remove dental plaque, including the use of disclosing agents (for example, Red Cote) to stain dental plaque in situ, and the correct use of a toothbrush and dental floss. Twice-daily tooth brushing with a fluoride-containing toothpaste (0.1 percent or 0.15 percent fluoride) and daily use of dental floss between all adjoining teeth are necessary. For patients with limited dexterity (for example, arthritis in the hands), electric toothbrushes, irrigators, or supplementary oral hygiene aids should be recommended.

DENTAL CARIES

Risk for an individual patient can be estimated from (1) the severity of past dental changes, (2) measurement of saliva flow rate and (3) estimation of caries-producing organisms in the saliva:

- Clinical signs of hyposalivation include: the presence of new or recurrent caries on root surfaces or incisal edges, sticky mucosal surfaces, absence of expressible saliva from the major salivary ducts, and absence of pooled saliva in the mouth floor.
- Measure unstimulated flow rate of whole saliva by having the patient empty saliva from their mouth into a graduated tube or preweighed container, while sitting in a forward-leaning position, for ten minutes. If flow is <1.0 ml/ten minutes, the patient is at much higher risk of caries.
- Kits permitting the culture and estimation of *Streptococcus mutans* in a dental office are commercially available (Dentocult SM Strip mutans test, Orion Diagnostica; Caries Screen SM, Apo Diagnostics). If the amount of salivary *S. mutans* exceeds 1×10^6 colony forming units/ml of whole saliva, prescribe a one-minute twice-daily rinse with 0.12 percent chlorhexidine (Peridex, PerioGard) for two weeks.

TOPICAL FLUORIDE

Topical Fluoride can be professionally applied and self-applied, in addition to the patient using a fluoride-containing dentrifice twice daily, as described above.

Professionally Applied

At dental office visits, a high-concentration agent can be applied, such as 1.23 percent acidulated phosphate fluoride gel or foam (many brands are available) for four minutes in a tray, or 2.25 percent fluoride varnish (Duraphat, Duraflor) directly onto the teeth. These applications can be repeated every six months, or more frequently if necessary.

Dental restoration. Restoration of carious lesions should use conservative intracoronal preparations. Light-cured glass ionomer cements should be used where practical, because they release fluoride and are more resistant to marginal decay. Note: subgingival margins and full coronal coverage should be avoided wherever possible for initial treatment of these patients. This is because subgingival margins are less accessible to topical fluoride, they are the usual site for recurrent caries, and caries there are more difficult to detect and to restore. Full veneer crowns, if ultimately necessary, should *not* be placed until caries are under complete control (that is, the patient has been free of new carious lesions for at least one year).

Recall examinations. At each recall visit, visual examination of dental surfaces should be supplemented with bitewing radiographs as needed, and the oral mucosa should be examined for signs of candidiasis (see below). The patient's dental plaque control should be reassessed by in vivo staining, and the importance of plaque control techniques should be reinforced. The amount of salivary *S. mutans* can be monitored and chlorhexidine rinse prescribed again as needed.

Self-Applied

Patients should be given specific instructions on the use of self-applied fluorides and their application demonstrated to the patient. The methods to be used depend on the severity of the patient's caries experience and/or the degree of salivary hypofunction:

- Patients at **low to moderate risk** of caries should use a 0.05 percent sodium fluoride rinse (available over-the-counter) for one to two minutes at least once daily, before sleep.

- Patients at **high risk** of caries should apply 1.1 percent neutral sodium fluoride gel (available only by prescription) in custom-made trays for five to ten minutes, daily. Patients should then floss between all teeth immediately after tray removal to carry fluoride to those adjoining dental surfaces. This is best done just before going to sleep.

ORAL CANDIDIASIS DIAGNOSIS AND TREATMENT

Diagnosis

About one third of patients with chronic hyposalivation develop oral candidiasis, usually of the chronic erythematous type, but usually not of the pseudomembranous type (thrush). Adequate treatment usually provides significant improvement of oral symptoms, in spite of continuing oral dryness.

Symptoms of chronic erythematous oral candidiasis include a burning sensation of the mucosa, intolerance to acidic or spicy foods, and a change in taste or development of a metallic taste. Some cases are asymptomatic.

Clinical signs of candidiasis include: (1) macular erythema on the dorsal tongue, palate, buccal mucosa, or denture-bearing mucosa, (2) atrophy of the filiform papillae on the dorsal tongue, or (3) angular cheilitis. The diagnosis can be confirmed by fungal culture of a swab specimen, from such a mucosal lesion, revealing significant numbers of colony-forming units of a *Candida* species, usually *C. albicans*.

Treatment

In patients with mild salivary hypofunction, this can be done easily with systemic drugs such as fluconazole. However, patients with severe chronic hyposalivation usually require the application of topical forms of polyene or imidazole antifungal drugs that *do not contain* sucrose or glucose, for periods of weeks or months (see table, page 163). Topical forms are necessary because systemically administered drugs do not reach the mouth of patients with severe hyposalivation in therapeutically adequate amounts. But topical drugs must not increase a patient's dental caries risk and, currently, all such "oral" antifungal drugs contain large amounts of glucose or sucrose that prevents a significant risk of supporting caries development in these patients.

Generally, the best topical antifungal drug for use in patients with severe hyposalivation and remaining natural teeth is nystatin vaginal tablets (which contain lactose but not sucrose or glucose). They must be dissolved slowly in the mouth for fifteen to twenty minutes, two or three times per day. Such patients will need frequent sips of water to allow the tablet to dissolve in that time.

For patients wearing partial or complete dentures, additional instructions and treatment are needed: (1) Dentures must be removed from the mouth before applying the antifungal drug. (2) Dentures must be disinfected by soaking overnight in a substance compatible with the denture material (for example, 1 percent sodium hypochlorite for dentures without exposed metal, or benzalkonium chloride diluted 1:750 in water for dentures with exposed metal) and rinsed carefully before reinserting in the mouth. (3) Nystatin topical powder may be applied on the fitting surface of a denture when it is reinserted in the mouth.

- **Treatment end-point.** Treatment should continue until the clinician has observed resolution of all the mucosal erythema, return of filiform papillae on the dorsal tongue, and resolution of associated oral symptoms.
- **Angular cheilitis.** The presence of angular cheilitis almost always indicates concurrent intraoral candidiasis. Angular cheilitis can be treated by nystatin or clotrimazole cream, but in most cases it should not be used without concurrently treating the intraoral infection, as described above.
- **Recurrence.** After treatment is completed, recurrence is fairly common and the patient must be retreated as described above. After one recurrence, re-treatment should be immediately followed by maintenance therapy (for example, continued use of half of a nystatin vaginal tablet slowly dissolved in the mouth each day, indefinitely).

SALIVARY FLOW STIMULATION

The following methods of stimulating salivary flow are effective, but only in those patients who retain some salivary function.

Physiological stimulation

Masticatory or gustatory stimuli, such as sugar-free chewing gum or sugar-free hard candies, can be used as needed to relieve oral symptoms. However, products marketed as "sugarless" actually contain some sugar and metabolizable carbohydrates, which are cariogenic; these products should not be used. Either method can provide an increase in salivary flow, but only while the stimulus is present in the mouth.

Pharmacological stimulation

Pharmacological stimulation can be provided by either of two currently available prescription drugs:

- Pilocarpine tablets (Salagen) can provide significantly increased salivary flow for one to two hours after systemic absorption. This drug should not be used in patients who have a history of uncontrolled asthma, acute iritis, or narrow-angle glaucoma. It may not be suitable for use by patients with unstable cardiovascular disease. Individual doses can be titrated, usually in the range between 5 mg tid and a maximum of 10 mg qid.
- Cevimeline (Evoxac), a newly released drug, provides similar flow rate stimulation, but may do so for a longer time per dose than pilocarpine. It has the same cautions as pilocarpine. Dosage is one 30 mg capsule, three times a day.

Use of Saliva Substitutes

Saliva substitutes can be helpful for patients with moderately severe chronic hyposalivation when used at bedside, while talking or while traveling. The glycerate polymer gel product appears to provide better reduction in dry mouth symptoms than CMC-based products, particularly in patients with severe xerostomia. None replace all the functions of natural saliva, none have long duration because they are swallowed, and none has been shown to prevent dental caries or oral candidiasis. Saliva substitutes are helpful, but only for patients with moderately severe and continuous hyposalivation, or those wearing a complete denture. There are several types of commercially available saliva substitutes:

- Carboxymethylcellulose (CMC)-based: (many brands)
- CMC-based with mucopolysaccharide: MouthKote (contains xylitol)
- Glycerate polymer gel: Oralbalance (contains xylitol)
- Mucin-based: Orthana (available only in Europe)

CURRENT PRESCRIPTION DRUG USE

A patient's current prescription drug use should be regularly reviewed to identify drugs whose principal or side effects contribute to decreased salivary function. If such drugs are being used, the problem should be discussed with the prescriber of the drug: it may be possible to eliminate the drug, replace it with another drug that has less effect on salivary function, or prescribe taking it at a less objectionable time (for example, in the evening instead of the morning).

Topical Antifungal Drugs for Treating Oral Candidiasis in Patients with Severe Hyposalivation*		
Drug and form	**Dose****	**Comments**
Nystatin vaginal tablets	2–4 tablets daily, 100,000 U / tablet	Dissolve each tablet slowly (15 minutes) in mouth using sips of water as necessary to aid dissolution[†]; has a medicinal taste; contains lactose.
Clotrimazole vaginal tablets	½ tablet twice daily, 100 mg / tablet	Dissolve slowly in mouth, as for nystatin vaginal tablets.[†] For use if there has been inadequate response to nystatin.
Nystatin cream	2–3 times daily, 100,000 U / gm	For treating angular cheilitis; usually must be used concurrently with an intraoral antifungal drug.
Nystatin topical powder	2 times daily, 100,000 U / gm	Apply a fairly even coating to the fitting surface of a clean, moistened denture; this supplements other intraoral antifungal drugs and may be helpful in maintenance therapy.

*Drugs selected on the basis of having little or no risk of supporting dental caries with prolonged use in patients with significant salivary hypofunction. All are unflavored. Candidiasis occurring in patients with normal salivary function or only mild hyposalivation can be usually be treated with systemic antifungal drugs, such as fluconazole.

**Duration of treatment for erythematous candidiasis in patients with salivary hypofunction ranges from about four weeks to several months (pseudomembranous oral candidiasis usually requires only one to two weeks of treatment).

†Patients wearing partial or complete dentures must remove them during this application to permit access of the drug to all mucosal surfaces. Dentures must be treated separately, as described in the text.

EXCESSIVE WATER CONSUMPTION

Patients need to understand that chronic hyposalivation is not associated with systemic dehydration; consuming large quantities of water does not overcome oral dryness. Frequent small sips of water during the day help reduce oral symptoms, but overuse may remove mucous coating the oral surfaces and further increase symptoms of dryness. Water consumption at night usually leads to sleep interruption from nocturia (excessive urination at night). Frequent sleep interruption usually leads to symptoms of fatigue. To avoid nocturia, patients should not drink water beginning one hour before sleep. Instead of drinking water during the night, a saliva substitute should be kept at bedside and used as necessary.

Resources

Chapter 1. Understanding Sjögren's Syndrome

The Sjögren's Syndrome Foundation
www.sjogrens.org
> The web site for the Sjögren's Syndrome Foundation, which is based in Baltimore, Maryland. The Sjögren's Syndrome Foundation offers information and support for patients, education for medical professionals, and advocacy for increased awareness of the disorder in the general public, media, and government. There are chat groups, help lines, and resources available to members.

The Arthritis Foundation
www.arthritis.org
> The central web site for information about arthritis and related conditions. There is a subsection about SjS in their diseases and conditions section, and a comprehensive overview of autoimmune conditions.

British Sjögren's Syndrome Association
http://ourworld.compuserve.com/homepages/bssassociation/
> This site provides helpful questions and answers about the symptoms and treatments of SjS.

The American Autoimmune Related Diseases Association
www.aarda.org
   This site is an excellent source for general autoimmune and specific SjS information.

Chapter 4. Dry Eyes

The American Medical Association
www.ama-assn.org/aps/amahg.htm
   American Medical Association has resources on their web site that will locate physicians who specialize in dry eye and SjS.

The American Optometric Association
www.aoanet.org
   This site has a "search" feature that allows you to search for an eye specialist.

Chapter 5. Dry Mouth, Nose, and Throat

The American Dental Association
www.ada.org
   The American Dental Association is a site of general interest with a good section on answers to commonly asked questions.

The American Dental Hygienists' Association
www.adha.org
   The American Dental Hygienists' Association answers specific questions about SjS.

Chapter 6. Extraglandular Involvement

The National Digestive Diseases Information Clearinghouse (NDDIC)
www.digestive.niddk.nih.gov
   The NDDIC is a service of the National Institute of Diabetes and Digestive and Kidney Diseases, part of the National Institutes of Health. Good site for information about digestive diseases and conditions such as constipation and celiac disease with links to other informative sites.

The Celiac Disease Foundation
www.celiac.org
   This site provides patient support and information along with links to
   other groups.

Interstitial Cystitis Association
www.ichelp.org
   Provides contact with the Interstitial Cystitis Association.

Irritable Bowel Syndrome Self Help and Support Group
www.ibsgroup.org
   An online resource for the IBS community.

Mind Body Digestive Center
www.mindbodydigestive.com
   This is a commercial organization that specializes in mind / body relationships of digestive diseases.

The Neuropathy Association
www.neuropathy.org
   Answers questions through an active chat line, provides hints, and links
   to membership in the Neuropathy Association.

The American Lung Association
www.lungusa.org

The American Academy of Dermatology
www.aad.org

Chapter 7. Pain and Fatigue

Centers for Disease Control
www.cdc.gov/ncidod/diseases/cfs/index.htm
   Link on the CDC's web site devoted to chronic fatigue syndrome.

American Pain Society
www.ampainsoc.org
   American Pain Society is an organization for practitioners and patients.

Helped launch American Pain Foundation (*www.painfoundation.org*), which is a nonprofit organization to help patients as information resource and advocacy center. This site has links to many other informative sites including those that help locate accredited pain clinics, physicians and therapists; information about alternative/complementary medicine; information about Medicare and Medicaid. They also offer online support for sufferers of pain.

American Chronic Pain Association
www.theacpa.org
Information, suggestions, and help for pain management.

American Academy of Pain Management
www.aapainmanage.org
American Academy of Pain Management has a patient information section. It is especially valuable as a source of links to other sites that may hold a particular interest for you.

Chapter 8. Special Considerations

The Sjögren's Syndrome Foundation
www.sjogrens.org
For access to the chat line about pregnancy, male patients, children, and other problems encountered by patients.

National Research Registry of Neonatal Lupus
www.msnyuhealth.org/hjd/hjd_search.jsp
This site is the registry at the Hospital for Joint Diseases in New York City that keeps track of affected mothers and children and fosters research into congenital heart block.

American Medical Association
www.ama-assn.org
The American Medical Association has complete lists of specialists.

The Arthritis Foundation
www.arthritis.org

The Arthritis Foundation has the most comprehensive, useful set of materials for people suffering from arthritic syndromes like SjS. They offer membership, an informative magazine, support groups, and web site.

The Scleroderma Foundation
www.scleroderma.org

Like other autoimmune disorder organizations, offers support through membership, support groups, magazine, and informative web site.

The Lupus Foundation of America
www.lupus.org

Lupus Around the World
www.mtio.com/lupus

Online forums and chat rooms for sufferers of lupus.

Fibromyalgia Network
www.fmnetnews.com

A fact- and suggestion-filled site for patients and one where you will find information and support.

Astroglide
www.astroglide.com

A web site with information about two products designed for vaginal dryness.

Chapter 9. The Emotional Toll of Chronic Disease

The Sjögren's Syndrome Foundation
www.sjogrens.org

Provides access to TalkSjo, the chat group for support and help; and SS-L, the chat group for information.

The National Mental Health Association
www.nmha.org
> Has information about emotional reactions, stress management and coping with loss. For specific help with depression, check out their depression screening site: *www.depression-screening.org*

The American Psychological Association
www.helping.apa.org
> Has a Help Center in which you can locate topics of interest to your work and home situation when dealing with emotional stress.

The National Institute of Mental Health
www.nimh.nih.gov/anxiety/anxietymenu.cfm
> Provides background on many emotional uncertainties; for anxiety.

The Arthritis Foundation
www.arthritis.org
> For many articles about the emotional toll of chronic disease.

Chapter 10. Medications for Sjögren's Syndrome

The Arthritis Foundation
www.arthritis.org
> A source for helpful, informative booklets, including the comprehensive publication, *Arthritis Today 2002 Drug Guide,* at no charge.

About.com
www.about.com
> An excellent, informative web site with information about health, including drugs and supplements. Their regular e-mailed newsletters are well written and reliable.

Medscape
www.medscape.com
> An exhaustive, complete medical information resource site.

U.S. Food and Drug Administration
www.fda.gov
> Drug information available through the Center for Drug Evaluation and Research.

Physicians Drug Reference
www.pdr.net
> Site listing of all drugs on the market with dosage, side effects, and contraindications for use by the public.

Medic Alert Foundation
www.medicalert.org
> Offers information and membership in the Medic Alert Foundation.

Chapter 12. Complementary Medicine

The Sjögren's Syndrome Foundation
www.sjogrens.org
> A fountainhead of information and assistance to sufferers.

National Center for Complementary and Alternative Medicine
www.nccam.nih.gov

Association of American Retired Persons
www.aarp.org/benefits-health/Articles/a2002-08-14-althealth
> Offers discounts on various alternative medical procedures—from massage to biofeedback—through their network of registered practitioners. The alternative medicine information on their web site is extensive and useful.

American Holistic Medical Association
www.holisticmedicine.org
> Check here for licensed physicians who practice integrative medicine.

For Your Self: Health
www.foryourselfhealth.com
> A medical practice of Dr. Amy Saltzman has information at her web site including six audiotapes of mindfulness meditation as we describe here.

American Academy of Medical Acupuncture
www.medicalacupuncture.org
(323) 937-5514

National Certification Commission for Acupuncture and Oriental Medicine
www.nccaom.org
(703) 548-9004

Biofeedback Certification Institute of America
www.bcia.org
(303) 420-2902

American Chiropractic Association
www.amerchiro.org
(703) 276-8800

International Chiropractors Association
www.chiropractic.org
(703) 528-5000

American Massage Therapy Association
www.amtamassage.org
(847) 864-0123

National Certification Board of Therapeutic Massage and Bodywork
www.ncbtmb.com
(703) 610-9015

American Yoga Association
www.americanyogaassociation.org
(941) 953-5859

Recommended Reading

Arthritis Today 2001 Supplement Guide, 67 Herbs, Vitamins and Other Natural Remedies by Judith Horstman. No charge. Available from the Arthritis Foundation at *www.arthritis.org* or (800) 207-8633.

Arthritis Foundation's Guide to Alternative Therapies by Judith Horstman ($24.95). An excellent compendium of alternative therapies.

The Chronic Pain Solution: Your Personal Path to Pain Relief: The Comprehensive, Step by Step Guide to Choosing the Best of Alternative and Conventional Medicine by James N. Dillard, M.D., D.C., C.Ac. (New York: Bantam Books, 2002). Another resource filled with information about complementary medicine techniques and resources.

Full Catastrophe Living by John Kabat-Zinn (New York: Dell Publishing, 1990).

Notes

Chapter 1. Understanding Sjögren's Syndrome

American Auto-immune Related Diseases Association (East Detroit, Mich.), 2002.

Chapter 2. Discovering a Diagnosis

Robert I. Fox, "Systemic Diseases Associated with Dry Eye," *International Ophthamological Clinics* 34 (Winter 1994): 71–87.

Chapter 3. You, Your Doctor, and Sjögren's Syndrome

B. Kane and D. Z. Sands, "Guidelines for the Clinical Use of Electronic Mail with Patients," *Journal of American Informatics Association* (January–February 1998): 1104–21.

B. Kane and D. Z. Sands, "Suggested Elements of a Patient-Provider Agreement for Electronic Communication," *Journal of American Informatics Association* (January–February 1998): 1104–21.

Mark E. Horowitz, "Doctor, You Have Mail," *The New York Times* (June 20, 2002), C3.

Chapter 4. Dry Eyes

R. M. Sullivan, J. M. Cermak, A. S. Papas, M. R. Dana, D. A. Sullivan, Schepens Eye Research Institute, Harvard Medical School, Brigham and Women's Hospital and Tufts University of Dental Medicine, MA, "Economic and Quality of Life Impact of Dry Eye Symptoms in Women with Sjögren's Syndrome," *Adv. Exp. Med. Biol.* (2002): 1183–8.

Winthrop University Hospital, Physician Education Program (Mineola, N.Y.), *Sjögren's Syndrome: New Insights and New Treatments* (2002).

Solomon et al., "Altered Cytokine Balance in the Tear Fluid and Conjunctiva of Patients with Sjögren's Syndrome Keratoconjunctiva Sicca," *Invest. Opthamol. Vis. Sc.* (2001): 201–11.

D. A. Sullivan, L. A. Wickham, E. M. Rocha, et al., "Androgens and Dry Eye in Sjögren's Syndrome," *Annuals of New York Academy of Science* (1999): 312–24.

P. Marsh and S. C. Pflugfelder, "Topical Nonpreserved Methylprednisolone Spray Therapy for Keratoconjunctiva Sicca in Sjögren's Syndrome," *Ophthamology* (April 1999): 811–16.

Perry Garber, "Eyelid Surgery for Patients with Dry Eye—Benefits and Pitfalls," *The Moisture Seekers Newsletter* (Winter 2000).

Gary H. Cassel, Michael D. Billig, and Harry G. Randall, *The Eye Book* (Baltimore, Md.: A Johns Hopkins Press Health Book, 1998).

F. Yamada, "Frontal Midline Theta Rhythm and Eye Blinking Activity During a VDT Task and Video Game: Useful Tools for Psychophysiology in Ergonomics," *Ergonomics* (1998): 678–88.

Chapter 5. Dry Mouth, Nose, and Throat

D. Mulherin et al., "Survey of Artificial Tear and Saliva Usage Among Patients with Sjögren's Syndrome," *Annals of Rheumatic Diseases* (2001): 1077–78.

Steven Carsons, Troy Daniels, Dena Reza, and Norman Talal, *Sjögren's Syndrome: New Insights and Treatments* (Winthrop University Hospital, 2001). A continuing education self-study aid on the diagnosis, treatment, and management of the patient with Sjögren's syndrome.

P. A. Johnstone, R. C. Niemtzow, and R. H. Riffenburgh, "Acupuncture for Xerostomia," *Cancer* (2002): 1151–66.

Devin J. Starlanyl and Mary Ellen Copeland, *The Fibromyalgia and Chronic Myofascial Pain Syndrome* (New Harbinger Publications, 1996).

F. B. Vivino, I. Al-Hashimi, Z. Kahn, et al., "Pilocarpine Tablets for the Treatment of Dry Eye and Dry Mouth Symptoms in Patients with Sjögren's Syndrome," *Arch. Intern. Med.* (1999): 174–81.

D. Petrone, J. J. Condemi, R. Fife, O. Gluck, et al. "A Double-Blind, Randomized Placebo-Controlled Study of Cevimeline in Sjögren's Syndrome Patients with Xerostomia and Keratoconjunctivitis Sicca," *Arthritis and Rheumatism* (2002): 745–54.

James Boyle, "The Digestive System and Sjögren's Syndrome," *Sjögren Digest,* special edition (National Sjögren's Syndrome Association, 1998).

K. Kawamata, H. Haraoka, S. Harohata, et al., "Pleurisy in Primary Sjögren's Syndrome," *Clin. Exp. Rheumatol.* (1997): 193–96.

M. Gyongosi, G. Pokorni, Z. Jabrik, et al., "Cardiac Manifestations in Primary Sjögren's Syndrome," *Ann. Rheum. Diseases* (1996): 450–54.

Chapter 7. Pain and Fatigue

A. Taddio, "Pain Management for Neonatal Circumcision," CDC guidelines in *Annals of Internal Medicine* (1994): 953–59.

Daniel J. Clauw, *Muskuloskeletal Signs and Symptoms of Fibromyalgia and Diffuse Pain Syndromes in Primer on Rheumatic Diseases,* 12th edition. (Atlanta: Arthritis Foundation, 2001).

The Moisture Seekers Newsletter (September 2002).

Chapter 8. Special Considerations

R. B. Rosenbaum, S. M. Campbell, and J. T. Rosenbaum, *Clinical Neurology of Rheumatic Diseases* (Butterworth-Heinemann, 1996).

W. H. Chen, J. H. Yeh, and H. C. Chiu, "Plasmapheresis in the Treatment of Ataxic Sensory Neuropathy Associated with Sjögren's Syndrome," *Eur. Neurology* (2001): 270–74.

F. Martinello, P. Fardin, M. Otyino, et al., "Supplemental Therapy in Isolated Vitamin E Deficiency Improves Peripheral Neuropathy and Prevents Progression of Ataxia," *Journal Neurological Science* (1998): 177–79.

M. D. Lockshin, E. Bonfa, K. Elkon, et al., "Neonatal Lupus Risk to Newborns of Mothers with Systemic Lupus Erythematosus," *Arthritis Rheumatology* (1998): 697–701.

Chapter 9. The Emotional Toll of Chronic Disease

Diagnostic and Statistical Manual of Emotional Disorders, 3rd edition (1987).

Chapter 10. Medications for Sjögren's Syndrome

T. Munster, J. P. Gibbs, et al., "Hydroxychloroquine Concentration-Response Relationships in Patients with Rheumatoid Arthritis," *Arthritis Rheumatology* (2002): 1460–69.

J. J. Palpoli and J. Waxman, "Colchicine Neuropathy or Vitamin B_{12} Deficiency Neuropathy," *New England Journal of Medicine* (1987): 1290–91.

R. W. Kuncl et al., "Colchicine Myopathy and Neuropathy," *New England Journal of Medicine* (1987): 1562–68.

M. R. Werbach, *Foundations of Nutritional Medicine* (Tarzana, Calif.: Third Line Press, 1997): 222–24.

S. D. Steinfeld, T. Appleboom, et al., "Treatment with Infliximab Restores Normal Aquaporin-5 Distribution in Minor Salivary Glands of Patients with Sjögren's Syndrome," *Arthritis Rheumatology* (2002): 2249–51.

J. A. Ship, P. C. Fox, et al., "Treatment of Primary Sjögren's Syndrome with Low-Dose Natural Human Interferon-Alpha Administered by the Oral Mucosal Route," *Journal Interferon Cytokine Research* (1999): 943–51.

Chapter 11. Nutrition and Autoimmune Disorders

J. M. Kremer, "Clinical Studies of Omega-3 Fatty Acid Supplementation in Patients Who Have Rheumatoid Arthritis," *Rheum. Dis. Clin.* (1991): 391–402.

N. Kromann and A. Green, "Epidemiological Studies in the Upernavik District, Greenland," *Acta Medica Scandinavica* (1980): 401–6.

W. C. Willett, *Eat, Drink and Be Healthy* (New York: Simon and Schuster, 2001).

O. Adams, "Anti-Inflammatory Diet in Rheumatic Diseases," *European Journal of Clinical Nutrition* (1995): 703–17.

R. J. Cousins, "Absorption, Transport and Hepatic Metabolism of Copper and Zinc," *Physiology Review* (1985): 238–43.

Ban Hock Toh, I. R. vanDriel, and P. A. Gleeson, "Pernicious Anemia," *New England Journal of Medicine* (1997): 1441–48.

Chapter 12. Complementary Medicine

Definition from the National Center for Complementary and Alternative Medicine (NCCAM), a component of the National Institutes of Health (NIH).

Budget of the United States Government, Fiscal Year 2003. Appendix, p. 444.

D. M. Eisenberg, R. C. Kessler, M. I. Van Roompay, et al., "Perceptions of Complementary Therapies Relative to Conventional Therapies Among Adults Who Use Both: Results From a National Survey," *Annals of Internal Medicine* (2001): 344–51.

Acupuncture, NIH Consensus Development Conference Statement, November 5–7, 1997.

C. Quinn, C. Chandler, and A. Moraska, "Massage Therapy and Frequency of Chronic Tension Headaches," *American Journal of Public Health* (2002): 1657–61.

K. Purstjarvu, O. Airaksinan, and P. J. Pontinen, "The Effect of Massage in Patients with Chronic Tension Headaches," *Acupuncture Electroth. Res.* (1990): 159–62.

J. Kabat-Zinn, E. Wheeler, T. Light, A. Skillings, M. Scharf, T. Cropley, D. Hosmer, and J. Bernard, "Influence of Mindfulness Meditation-Based Stress Reduction Intervention on Rates of Skin Clearing in Patients with Moderate to Severe Psoriasis Undergoing Phototherapy (UVB) and Photochemotherapy (PUVA)," *Psychosomatic Medicine* (1998): 625–32.

J. Kabat-Zinn, L. Lipworth, and R. Burney, "The Clinical Use of Mindfulness Meditation for the Self-Regulation of Chronic Pain," *Journal of Behavioral Medicine* 8, no. 2 (1985).

J. Kabat-Zinn and A. Chapman-Waldrop, "Compliance with an Outpatient Stress Reduction Program: Rates and Predictors of Program Completion," *Journal of Behavioral Medicine* 11, no. 4 (1988).

J. Kabat-Zinn, L. Lipworth, R. Burney, and W. Sellers, "Four-Year Follow-Up of a Meditation-Based Program for the Self-Regulation of Chronic Pain: Treatment Outcomes and Compliance," *Clinical Journal of Pain* (1987).

J. Kabat-Zinn, "An Outpatient Program in Behavioral Medicine for Chronic Pain Patients Based on the Practice of Mindfulness Meditation: Theoretical Considerations and Preliminary Results," *General Hospital Psychiatry* (1982): 33–47.

B. Hellman, M. Budd, J. Borysenko, D. McClelland, and H. Benson, "A Study of the Effectiveness of Two Group Behavioral Medicine Interventions for Patients with Psychosomatic Complaints," *Behavioral Medicine* (1990): 165–73.

Afterword

S. Winer, I. Astsaturov, R. Cheung, H. Trui, et al., "Primary Sjögren's Syndrome and Deficiency of ACA69," *The Lancet* (2002): 10063.

T. Maruta, R. C. Colligan, et al., "Optimists vs. Pessimists: Survival Rate among Medical Patients over a 30-year Period," *Mayo Clinic Proc.* (2000): 140–43.

C. Peterson, M. E. Seligman, and G. E. Vaillant, "Pessimistic Explanatory Style Is a Risk Factor for Physical Illness. A Thirty-five-Year Longitudinal Study," *J. Pers. Soc. Psychol.* (1998): 23–27.

Index